THE FATBURN FIX

Also by Catherine Shanahan, M.D.

Deep Nutrition

Food Rules

THE FATBURN FIX

*Boost Energy, End Hunger,
and Lose Weight by
Using Body Fat for Fuel*

Catherine Shanahan, M.D.

FLATIRON
BOOKS
NEW YORK

This book contains the opinions and ideas of its author. It is intended to provide helpful general information on the subjects that it addresses. It is not in any way a substitute for the advice of the reader's own physician(s) or other medical professionals based on the reader's own individual conditions, symptoms, or concerns. If the reader needs personal medical, health, dietary, exercise, or other assistance or advice, the reader should consult a competent physician and/or other qualified health care professionals. The author and publisher specifically disclaim all responsibility for injury, damage, or loss that the reader may incur as a direct or indirect consequence of following any directions or suggestions given in the book or participating in any programs described in the book.

To open minds and gentle hearts

Contents

THE FATBURN FIX

Introduction

Fix Your Fatburn, Fix Your Health

THE FAT TRAP

Claudia was a twenty-seven-year-old bookkeeper and mother of two with a weight problem. In college, she'd gain a few pounds after holiday parties and trips, but she'd quickly get back to normal weight by cutting down her portion sizes and going to the gym. After her second baby, however, that strategy wasn't working. In spite of cutting soda and working with a trainer, it was all she could do to keep the weight gain trajectory from climbing higher and higher.

Carl was a thirty-two-year-old software engineer, high school basketball coach, and first-time dad who thought he was in perfect health—until a workplace wellness screening uncovered high blood pressure and low HDL cholesterol levels. His doctor told him he needed to lose weight and buy a prescription that Carl was hesitant to take, so he wanted my opinion on the best way forward.

Cathy was a forty-six-year-old music teacher whose doctor told her losing 10 pounds would help to control her blood pressure. She came to me deeply depressed. After exercising regularly for six months, following a program of protein shakes, salads, and lean meat, she had managed to lose weight. Nevertheless her last round of blood work showed she was now prediabetic. "I worked so hard to do everything right. What's wrong with me?" she asked, near tears in a broken voice.

Cindy was sixteen and had been overweight since she was eight. She'd just found out her irregular, painful periods were due to polycystic ovarian disease, and her mother brought her to me hoping there was something Cindy could do besides take birth control pills to fix her hormone problems.

Charlie was sixty-four and planning to retire next year. He came to me after the shock of his life. What seemed like a bout of his usual heartburn landed him in the hospital with a diagnosis of a "minor" heart attack. Now he had a stent and four new prescriptions. He'd never been particularly concerned about his weight or his diet, although he knew both were unhealthy, but now he was worried he wouldn't be around to enjoy his grandchildren.

These are just a few examples of the kinds of folks I see all day, every day in my medical practice. And while it may seem as if they each have different problems, the reality is their stories are all rooted in the same common soil: they've lost their ability to burn body fat for fuel. Our ability to burn body fat is an underappreciated gift of nature and an unrecognized requirement for metabolic health that we almost never think about—until it starts to slip away.

Losing the ability to burn body fat traps you in a downward spiral of reduced energy, increased hunger—which drives overeating—and slowly worsening health.

You might assume you can burn body fat just fine, or at least you could if you got into a good diet and exercise routine. But what most people don't know is that exercising rarely restores your ability to burn body fat to its full capacity. What's more, most diets out there will make blocked fatburn even worse.

Let me repeat that. Most diets actually damage your metabolism further. Not only does this set you up for weight regain once you complete the diet, it can also cause entirely new health problems you never had before.

I've seen it time and again. People follow any number of diets that have worked for them in the past, diets that successfully enabled them to lose 10, 20, even 30 pounds or more. At some point, having regained that weight again, they'll try the same routine, still thinking they're doing all the right things. But this time, their body won't respond the same way. The pudge refuses to budge.

And that's often when people notice other new health problems developing. Patients often repeat the very same phrase to me: "It's like my body is starting to fall apart." You may be diagnosed with prediabetes, like Cathy the music teacher was, or thyroid disease or another hormone problem—or even an autoimmune disease. Alternative practitioners often discuss adrenal fatigue or candida. When treatments for these conditions fail to provide the hoped-for results, many people get an inkling that there's still something else going on that nobody has yet discovered. That's what this book is about.

The reality is that today's gold-standard dietary advice has caused your metabolic problems. As you've followed the advice, your metabolism has become increasingly dysfunctional, and less able to do its number one job: *supply your cells with energy.*

Energy is the basis of health. When your energy declines, you change how you think and behave—ever so gradually that you may not be able to pinpoint when it began. Your energy-deprived brain becomes relatively less capable of dealing with emotional stress, problem solving, and planning. You may grow hungrier and prone to overeating. You may be less interested in activity and exercise. You can even experience difficulty with basic body functions like digestion, blood flow regulation, sleep, and hormone balance—all of which require energy. The list of over-the-counter or prescription medications starts to grow.

Experience has taught me that blocked fatburn is more than just an inconvenience that makes you feel bad and gain weight. It puts you on course to develop type 2 diabetes—a disease that's now taking over the country. Type 2 diabetes is not just a problem of high blood sugar, as we commonly believe. It's a disease that develops as your body loses its ability to use fat for fuel. It's also a disease that multiplies your risk of hospitalization, causing dangerously high blood pressure, nerve damage, learning and memory problems, joint degeneration, failure to eliminate toxins, skin diseases, heart attacks, heart failure, kidney failure, liver disease, strokes, and even cancer. There's no part of your body—no tissue, organ, or metabolic function—that is immune from complications of type 2 diabetes, which is to say there's no part of you that blocked fatburn leaves untouched.

Fortunately, just as our metabolism crumbles under the influence of a terrible diet, it begins to heal the moment we set our diets right. Just as we can lose this metabolic ability to convert body fat into cellular energy, we can also gain it back. Doing so will not only enable you to lose weight and keep it off for good; it will greatly improve and extend your life.

ESCAPE THE WEIGHT LOSS AND REGAIN CYCLE

When I first trained in clinical medicine nearly thirty years ago, weight was thought to be mainly a cosmetic problem, not something that shortened your life. The only accepted complications of being overweight were excessive wear and tear on the joints and skin conditions as a result of moisture retention in body creases. Obesity was something doctors like me would see just a few times a month, and it was mostly a concern for women— many men seemed to enjoy being larger.

Decades later, it's widely accepted that most chronic disease is associated with obesity, and that losing weight can help alleviate suffering and sickness of all kinds. Still, even though it's clear how important it is for many people to lose weight, we're not very good at helping to get the job done.

In my early days as a physician, I was not much help either. The best I could do for someone who was stuck in their overweight body was to check their thyroid, a simple blood test that would nearly always come back normal, and then offer a prescription for an appetite suppressant. Seems pretty limited, right? Well, it was. Although I decided to become a doctor with the goal of getting to the underlying cause of health problems, medical school didn't always encourage us to get to the real root causes of our patients' conditions. This left me with a hollow feeling and a sense that there were some missing pieces of the puzzle still out there for me to find.

I found the first of many missing pieces on a Hawaiian island. In Hawaii, the longest-lived state, folks in their fifties and sixties were often healthier than their own children and grandchildren. This was of particular interest to me because in my own family, all three of my siblings also had health problems that no one in the family had faced before. I began to see what had happened to my family as part of a much larger pattern of children developing new illnesses that they were not genetically predisposed to. But I had no clue what was behind it. In 2001, shortly after I too developed a health problem, I began to understand that the root cause of this pattern had always been right in front of me, in the food I was eating.

The desperate need to heal myself forced me to face a reality I'd been blinded to for many years: nearly everything I'd learned about nutrition in medical school was wrong. In fact, most people dishing out dietary advice don't actually learn much about nutrition. This includes your typical dietitians, sports nutritionists, trainers, chiropractors, and naturopathic doctors, as well as medical doctors trained at well-respected institutions. Most health practitioners give terrible nutrition advice because most of the nutrition education they receive during training is either exactly backwards or just plain wrong.

That was no easy thing to accept, and in my first book, *Deep Nutrition*, my husband and I wrote about the many avenues of inquiry we pursued to buck the medical orthodoxy and determine what a healthy human diet really looks like. We exposed the evidence that nutrient-poor food affects how symmetrical we look, how well we grow, and how well we age, and concluded that traditional fats like butter and coconut oil have been wrongly convicted for crimes committed by vegetable oils and sugars.

In the years after *Deep Nutrition* was published, I traveled the country visiting the best weight loss clinics from coast to coast. These clinics were run by MDs who had dedicated their careers to helping people lose weight and were now skilled practitioners, adept at choosing from a variety of tools at their disposal, including appetite suppressants, ready-to-eat meal programs, low-carb diets, mind-body approaches, stress reduction, and exercise. The treatment approaches were agreed upon between doctor and patient in conversations that lasted up to an hour at times. And the programs initially worked well for many happy patients. The treatment approaches had all converged around creating fast weight loss right out of the gate in order to keep people motivated.

But it wasn't all success stories. When people did not lose weight as fast as they expected, they dropped out of the program. Other folks who did lose weight quickly developed complications, including gallstones and gout. And a number of people developed diabetes even while following the program. It was as if they were being doubly punished. Not only did all the work they did to lose the weight rapidly evaporate, their metabolic health had taken a turn for the worse. That was when I began to suspect there may be something fundamentally wrong with the lose-weight-fast-and-keep-folks-motivated strategy.

The nail in the coffin hit home while visiting a longstanding medical weight loss practice, where the doctor had been in the community for nearly thirty years, graphically tracking his loyal patients' weights and ages in yellowed paper charts. Over and over I saw the same pattern in their records: a line plummeting down dramatically, then plateauing, then shooting up again. Up and down, up and down, over and over and over, recording weight gains and losses over the years in an upward-trending zigzag. Each peak of this zigzagging line was inevitably higher than the last, representing a new maximum weight. Each dip was higher as well, as achieving ideal weight became an ever more impossible-seeming goal.

My critical insight during these years of study came while listening to a patient, a mother of two who worked full-time. She used the words "too tired" about fifty times during the encounter. She said she could only muster up the energy to make dinner after a candy bar—or other snack—she'd pick up at the dollar store on the way home. It wasn't just her. I started noticing that patient after patient was eating, drinking, snacking, and otherwise using food to boost their energy.

In all the physiology books I'd ever read, I'd learned that eating is actually supposed to make us slightly drowsy so that we can digest our food in restful peace. But what I was hearing was that people were more fatigued a few hours after meals than they were immediately after eating. It seemed to me that something very important was happening that nobody was addressing. I began to consider how the obesity epidemic might be tied to this pattern.

Feeling energized right after eating and then feeling fatigued a few hours later can lead a person to believe that they're tired because they've just burned up all the calories in their last meal. And that would lead a person to believe that if they want to get more energy, they need to eat again—some kind of snack or energizing beverage, like an apple or soda.

While that line of thinking seems reasonable enough, it's totally wrong. We're supposed to be able to use our *body fat* for energy between meals. That's why we have body fat! We're not supposed to need regular snacks—or even regular meals. We're supposed to feel fine eating just one meal a day if we so choose, as long as we meet our nutritional needs in that one sitting.

BURNING BODY FAT VERSUS DIETARY FAT

Burning body fat is not the same thing as burning dietary fat. Burning body fat refers to burning off the flab you want to get rid of. Burning dietary fat refers to burning off a few of the fat calories from a recent meal.

The two processes are very different. Anyone who eats fat can burn some of that just-consumed fat once it hits their circulation, no matter how healthy or unhealthy their metabolism. But if your body fat is full of the unusual fatty acids in vegetable oils, those unusual fatty acids in your body fat slowly but surely damage your cells. In an attempt to slow the damage, your metabolism slowly but surely makes a seismic shift from relying mostly on body fat for energy between meals to relying mostly on sugar for energy between meals.

Throughout the book, I'll be using the term "fatburn" to refer specifically to your body's ability to burn body fat and the term "burning fat" to refer specifically to burning dietary fat.

I began to realize that the problem of obesity is not driven by simply eating too much or not exercising enough. It is driven by feeling hungry and tired too often. That hunger and fatigue reflects a serious metabolic problem. And the serious problem is that your body fat has grown less and less capable of serving up energy to your cells.

In other words, if you are struggling with your weight, it's because you are no longer able to stave off hunger and support your energy by burning your body fat.

The resulting energy deficits have a cascading effect on every aspect of your metabolism, including your hormones, your appetite, your arterial health, and your memory and moods. In order to lose weight and keep it off for good, you must repair the broken elements of your metabolism. You must fix your fatburn.

WHAT BLOCKS FATBURN?

To fix your fatburn, you have to understand what "broke" it.

The problem of obesity is not new. The proportion of the population affected by obesity is the issue. In the 1800s and early 1900s, obesity rates were remarkably steady and low, estimated in the 1 to 2 percent range. Rates climbed noticeably for the first time shortly after World War I, then fell during the Great Depression, then picked up pace after World War II. In the 1980s, however, the epidemic began in earnest, with rates climbing at least a percentage point or two every year on a nearly continuous basis, to reach nearly 40 percent by 2015–16.

What has fueled the last few decades of obesity rate expansion?

Most obesity researchers point, correctly, to an influential set of guidelines titled "Nutrition and Your Health: Dietary Guidelines for Americans, 1980." The government document encouraged Americans to cut down their intake of saturated fat. Restaurants, processed food manufacturers, and home chefs pulled back on their use of the traditional fats like butter and coconut oil—but of course when you use less of something, you necessarily use more of something else. And here's where my thinking diverges from most obesity researchers'.

While many excellent writers and physicians have pointed out that between 1970 and 1994, the average US adult's total carbohydrate intake jumped from about 200 grams per day to about 260, where it more or less has stayed since, I don't think it's just about the carbs.

Yes, the average person did start eating more carbs, especially the kind of carbohydrate we call sugar. But there's a detail about the fat consumption that often gets lost in the arguments. Fat consumption consistently hovered around 80 grams per person per day in spite of the reduction in butter, coconut oil, and other saturated-fat-rich foods.

How could that be? How could it be that we cut back our saturated fat intake but yet continue eating the same amount of fat, roughly an average of 80 grams of fat per day?

The answer lies in realizing that the terms "fat" and "saturated fat" do not mean the same thing. "Saturated fat" is actually a chemical term that refers to a type of fatty acid present in higher proportion in certain kinds of foods. So when you hear that we cut back on saturated fat, that does not mean we cut back on all fats. What we did was make a fat exchange.

We exchanged one kind of fat for another. And that has made all the difference.

In *Deep Nutrition* I described how this fat exchange has increased our consumption of something called *vegetable oils*. We are going to learn more about these little-known oils very soon. What I want you to know now is that when we consume large enough volumes of the vegetable oils, they can promote inflammation. *Deep Nutrition* detailed how the fatty acids in vegetable oils are chemically unstable, making them pro-inflammatory and capable of causing heart attacks, strokes, brain diseases, and more. What I've learned since *Deep Nutrition*, and what you'll come to understand as you continue, is that these same oils also promote carbohydrate addiction at the cellular level.

In other words, the kind of fat you eat changes what kinds of fuel your body's cells can use, which determines everything about your health.

The most dangerous piece of nutritional advice that medical professionals give hinges around fats.

To comply with the 1980s-era nutrition guidelines, healthcare practitioners have been telling people to cut down on animal-based saturated fats and replace them with vegetable oils, also known as seed oils and RBD oils (refined bleached deodorized). Today, the majority of meat and dairy available in grocery stores is low-fat or fat-free. We *are* eating much less animal-based saturated fat than we were just a generation ago, and clearly that has not led to a decrease in obesity. (Apparently our health experts are oblivious to this reality because they're still blaming saturated fat for the ever increasing rates of obesity and chronic disease.)

While most grocery store foods are much lower in saturated fats today than they were in 1970, they are much higher in vegetable oils. We are now consuming historically high volumes of vegetable oils. And it's high time we consider how these unusual fats damage your metabolism.

I've discovered that when a person's diet is composed of extraordinary amounts of these unusual fats, their body will be composed of extraordinary amounts of these same unusual fats. As you will come to appreciate, this unusual body composition is the reason that your body cannot currently use

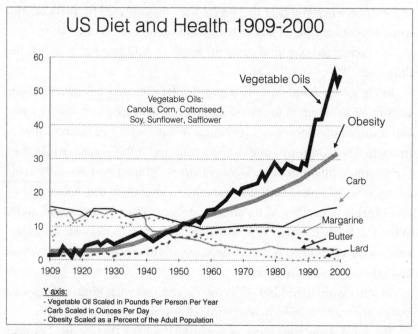

This chart tells the whole story. As we've eaten more vegetable oils, we've gotten fatter. Since 1909 we've not made a significant increase in our butter, lard, margarine, or carb consumption. Gluten consumption has not changed much, as reflected (roughly) by the relatively flat carb-consumption line. But throughout the century, the more vegetable oil we ate, the fatter and sicker we became as a nation.

body fat to suppress your hunger or fuel all the myriad daily activities an ordinary body must do.

So if your body fat can't readily supply your daily energy needs, then how do you function at all?

That's where sugar comes in. When your body fat stores no longer serve to energize your body's cells, then your metabolism immediately starts gearing up to burn sugar instead. You don't feel this when it first starts happening, but it represents a fundamental change in how your body operates.

The more your cells are forced to depend on sugar, the faster you'll develop a complicated set of unhealthy habits that you may not be aware you have. These habits will include seeking out foods high in sugar and starch. Sugar dependence also impairs your hormone function, so you become more prone to storing body fat and highly resistant to burning it off. Your body's organs will be forced to wage war against one another for access to energy. Your health will continually progress down a path you don't want to take—the road to chronic disease and disability.

FIXING YOUR FATBURN

There is one way to escape the sugar-dependency cycle and restore your health. You will have to lose your attachment to the typical goal of a weight loss book, namely your weight. You will learn to focus instead on an entirely new goal—the energy you will gain. Energy is going to be your saving grace. Fixing your fatburn is the only way to end sugar dependency and escape the metabolic trap you've fallen into because burning your body fat is the only way to provide your body the energy it constantly craves. Fixing your fatburn as fast and safely as possible, using all-natural foods and a few other metabolic "hacks," is the goal of this book.

Part One: Achieve Your True Health Potential

In Part One of the book, we'll discover how restoring your ability to burn body fat can give you enough energy to dramatically improve your quality of life. After a few months on the plan, most of my patients tell me they can't believe how much better they feel, how their extra energy has translated into more time, and how much more they're able to accomplish. They can accomplish so much more because, instead of using willpower to fight off daily hunger pangs, they've used it to create new, healthy habits.

Understanding the power of habit is key. Most folks I've worked with are shocked to discover how their current habits have slowly shifted over the years to the point they eat without actually realizing they're doing it! You'll learn how habits can hide behaviors, making them invisible to your conscious mind. You may be shocked at what you find when you become more conscious of your daily eating routines. After following the plan for just a few months, most folks are pleasantly surprised to discover how much more they enjoy the wider variety of foods that they've learned to include in their new daily routines. To get you to that happy place, this book will help you create brand-new eating habits.

Part Two: Meet Your Metabolism

Part Two is where we'll take a deep dive into your metabolism and look at the scientific processes that lead to blocked fatburn. You'll learn that the ability to generate energy from your body fat depends on four separate metabolic systems that exist within your body. You will learn how each of the four is shaping your day-to-day experiences, how all four systems must work together in a cooperative way, and how repairing damage to each is going to make your life so much easier. I'll also give you tools that will to allow you to assess the degree of damage in each of your four fatburn systems, which will help you determine how best to boost your ability to burn body fat.

At the end of this part you will assess the health of each of your four fatburn systems, using the Fatburn Factor quiz. The result of the quiz is a score, a number from 0 to 100, that assesses your body's ability to convert fat to energy. You will use your Fatburn Factor score to pinpoint the amount of damage you have in each of the four fatburn systems, which helps you to better appreciate how your struggles with weight, hunger, and fatigue are all going to be put to rest by following the plan.

Part Three: The Fatburn Fix Plan

Part Three of the book takes everything we've learned and combines that knowledge into a step-by-step guide covering what, exactly, you need to do in order to burn your body fat. First, we will lay out the five core rules to fix your fatburn. Then, we will teach you how the first phase of the Fatburn Fix Plan will prepare you for the second.

The first phase of the plan is what makes this approach unique. Unlike other diets that introduce radical changes and encourage radically rapid weight loss, this plan focuses on preparing your metabolism to lose weight first, before teaching you how to go about losing weight in a sustainable, even enjoyable way.

During Phase I you will shift your foods from those that provide energy briefly to those that provide energy for much longer. Instead of the sugars and starches that only give you short bursts of energy, you'll learn about carbohydrate-containing foods and healthy fats that sustain your energy for much longer. Many people choose to follow a keto-style diet during this phase, but it's not necessary to continually cut carbs to that degree—as you'll learn.

By the time you are ready for Phase II, you will have repaired your metabolism to the point that you can stop relying on food to sustain your energy between meals and start relying on your body fat—like nature intended. In Phase II, you'll be restricting the number of meals you eat per day to just one or two, depending on your preference.

My goal when developing the plan was to make it sustainable. You will learn about specific foods that support your mental clarity—and mental clarity makes learning and change much easier. You won't need to cook every meal from scratch, spend your life wishing you could eat forbidden foods, or do any more exercise than you already do. You will be given fast meal ideas and all the flavors you crave. You will not be told you need to eat foods that you don't enjoy. You will be given choices of new foods to experience. You will not be forced to push your way through it on willpower alone.

I want you to stay on this program for life. I want to make it as easy as possible for you to follow the plan even when life circumstances are stressful, chaotic, and otherwise far from ideal. No diet will work if you can only follow it some of the time. That's why I'll teach you to use healthy shortcut foods that taste delicious and can save you precious time.

WHAT MAKES THIS PROGRAM DIFFERENT?

If you've worked with a dietitian or read diet books in the past, you will find this program very different. It's different because, first and foremost, it focuses on the right goal: giving you energy. Weight loss is not the right goal—not until you have more energy and you experience less hunger. The first phase serves to give you more energy and control your hunger, laying the groundwork to make weight loss effortless and lasting. You may lose weight in either phase, but Phase II is where the focus shifts to losing weight.

This approach is the opposite of most other diets. Most programs focus on rapid weight loss in order to get you started. But that's a problem because it means your ability to feel good about yourself is entirely dependent on what happens when you step on a scale or slip on a certain pair of jeans. And that's not right. I want you to feel good about yourself because you have discovered how to be a more energetic person. When we're motivated mainly by weight loss, it's hard to keep the motivation alive when your weight plateaus, and besides, I want you to be motivated by something more important. I don't want you to focus on external factors like the number on your bathroom scale. Instead, I'm going to teach you how to gauge your metabolic recovery based on how much better you are feeling. This approach teaches you the awareness you need to radically change your relationship with food and radically improve your health.

In other words, the Fatburn Fix is not about depriving yourself to shrink by five dress sizes in time for your daughter's wedding. Instead, it's about restoring normal appetite so that you actually crave healthy foods. Nor is the Fatburn Fix about impressing your high school classmates with your tiny waistline at the next reunion—and then ballooning back up again after you fall back into old patterns. Rather, it's about impressing them with glowing skin, mental balance, and the energy you bring to the room—and then looking even younger the following year (because you will!).

Importantly, the Fatburn Fix is not about outthinking your metabolism. It's about cooperating with your metabolism so you can gain health as you lose weight. It's also not about setting the alarm extra early to do a workout. It's about balancing hormones, normalizing your blood sugar, and improving organ function.

The Fatburn Fix is certainly not all about a single sound bite solution like cutting carbs or eating only plants or just meat. It is about learning to feed yourself with wholesome fresh or freshly prepared foods, the way people have for millennia. It's about giving you a deeper understanding of how your body works so you can focus on the right goals and develop the habits you need to fully heal yourself and inspire those you care about to do the same.

JOIN THE FATBURN FAMILY

Over the past decade I've worked with well over a thousand patients, helping them not just to lose weight but also to recover from nearly every chronic, recurring medical condition in the book. Some of these recoveries have been truly miraculous.

I'm talking about patients like the eighty-year-old diabetic diagnosed with esophageal cancer who, after radiation and chemo had minimal effect on his tumor size, elected to try the Fatburn program. He was so motivated to follow the program to a T that, in spite of being a diabetic for decades, he got off his insulin and other diabetes drugs over a weekend and then went on to shrink his cancerous tumor to the point it was invisible on a PET scan just ten weeks later. Another story comes from the fifty-five-year-old Napa Valley winemaker headed for bilateral knee replacements who instead lost fifty pounds and is now running half marathons. And another from a sixty-five-year-old retired pilot with diabetes and crippling leg cramps due to poor circulation who was told his only option was arterial bypasses. After following the plan for six months, he shocked his would-be surgeon by getting off diabetes medications and is now walking three miles a day. Another happy story comes from a thirty-three-year-old female graphic designer with insulin resistance and abnormally high testosterone who'd failed in vitro fertilization six times. Now, several years later and still following the plan, she has delivered two healthy babies, completely naturally. These are just the tip of the iceberg; there are many, many more stories out there, and even more waiting to be told.

This book will give you the tools you need to experience the same incredible turnarounds I've witnessed in my clinic. Thanks to the work of dedicated researchers around the world, we now know more than we ever did before about the power we have to reclaim control of our health. With this book, I've compiled the best, most pertinent research for you, along with my own work, into a simple, streamlined set of directions. These instructions will enable you to do so much more than lose weight. You no longer need to stumble forward on your own, hoping you run into the right set of solutions on a journey through the internet that may or may not reveal the answers you need. The science of converting body fat to fuel has arrived. Now let's put it to use.

Part One

ACHIEVE YOUR
TRUE HEALTH POTENTIAL

The Fatburning Advantage: More Energy

Get the Energy You Need to Lose the Fat You Don't

IN THIS CHAPTER YOU'LL LEARN

- When your metabolism is damaged, you lack energy.
- When you lack energy, you want to eat more often, and most of us seek out foods that make metabolic damage worse.
- It's a trap—but you can escape if you can get more energy.

ENERGY SHAPES YOUR TEMPERAMENT

Are you a morning person, or do you need a few hours to really get going each day? Does a long day at work make you want to head outside for a walk or take a nap? Do you jump out of your seat with excitement when you get an idea about something fun to do, or do you sit quietly in place? Do you find that when you're really hungry certain people, or certain tasks, irritate you a lot more than they do when you've had something to eat?

Believe it or not, your answers to these questions depend less on your personality than they do on the health of your *metabolism*. So an unhealthy metabolism not only impairs your energy; it also impairs your ability to attain your full human potential.

First, let's define metabolism: your metabolism provides your body with energy. A healthy metabolism supports pretty much everything your body does, because every physiologic function relies on energy production, everything from learning, memory, and motivation to DNA replication, to cell division, to hormonal function, to the replacement of old worn-out tissue with new growth, to the removal of toxic materials from the body.

A healthy metabolism uses body fat to sustain your energy all day so that you don't need to rely on food to keep your energy up. When your metabolism is healthy, you have plenty of energy all day long even if you don't have time to eat. You don't need to snack when you can burn your body fat. You don't need beverages to keep you focused. When your metabolism is healthy, your body naturally stays at a healthy weight because your body fat provides you with energy that makes you enjoy staying active.

The important point here is that the job of your metabolism is to ensure all your cells have all the energy they need all the time. When your metabolism is unable to do its job properly, your energy drags. When your energy drags, it affects your moods, your relationships, your interest in exercise, and your ability to function at work. It even impairs your libido, affecting your interest in sex.

Low energy also makes you gain weight. When your energy is down, you're going to feel lazier than when your energy is up. You're more likely to choose the elevator over the stairs, and you're not likely to want to cook a healthy meal from scratch after a long day. All the reduced activity reduces your calorie needs, which makes it all too easy for your portion sizes to exceed the reduced amount of calories you need.

Worse, many people with low energy start using food to keep their energy levels up. They start to use snacks and beverages here and there throughout the day to help sustain their energy. They may need to take snack breaks at work to stay focused on the job. They start to eat slightly larger meals, hoping to prevent the need for snacks. Or they may be so hungry by mealtimes that they eat with their eyes, piling on more than they need or getting second helpings when they know they've already had enough. All the extra snacking and mealtime portioning can add up to a lot of calories, which makes you prone to gaining weight. It also makes cutting calorie intake—and thus forcing your reluctant metabolism to burn body fat—feel like physical torture, or at least feel like a lot more work than it should.

Everyone with a weight problem developed their condition due in large part to disruptions in cellular energy supply that slowly but surely over the years cause ever more widespread metabolic damage. What I'm saying is your metabolic damage began *before* you gained weight, not afterward. It is the reason you gained weight, not just a consequence of the weight gain.

Because metabolic damage is the cause of weight gain, rather than simply a consequence of weight gain, this means that correcting a weight problem is more complicated than instructing you to eat less and exercise more. For one thing, that's not easy to do while you don't have the energy you need to make it possible. In order to lose weight, you have to restore your metabolic ability to supply your body's cells with energy so you can stop needing to snack, stop overportioning at meals, and start to be more active. If your body can produce enough energy, you'll be less hungry and less tempted by snacks that may be lying around. You'll be less prone to overfilling your plate. You'll also be more energized and ready to get up and be active. All those happy consequences of ample cellular energy practically guarantee you'll lose weight. That's how a healthy eating program that heals your metabolism (as opposed to causing more metabolic damage) is going to make your weight loss permanent.

So where will that newfound energy come from? When you follow the Fatburn Fix Plan, your energy will come first from foods that sustain your energy and then later, in Phase II, from your ultimate source of supercharged energy: body fat.

BODY FAT IS FULL OF ENERGY

Most of the time when we talk about body fat, we're thinking about weight. But the fact is, we're actually talking about energy. Body fat is full of energy. And when we talk about fat as energy, suddenly everything changes. We're not talking about what we look like; we're talking about how we feel. Do we feel good? Do we feel confident? Do we feel like getting our work done, cleaning the house, going to school, making a difference in the world?

If you woke up energized, in a good mood, and had enough energy all day to check off everything on your need-to-do list, imagine how much that could improve your self-confidence. If you had the mental energy to quickly resolve problems or sidestep arguments or brighten someone's day with a surprise gift, imagine how much that could improve your entire outlook on life. Our body fat is designed to be the steady source of energy that lasts all day if we need it to, or even longer. Nature designed our bodies to be able to go between meals without energy dips whether the time between meals is two hours or twenty or even more.

In other words, our body fat is supposed to free us up from the need to constantly think about food so we can focus on living life.

But these days, our body fat does not do this. At least not for most of us. And this is the key point of the book, the result of decades of working with patients and researching how foods affect our health. The shocking truth is that modern body fat is very different than what nature intended. The difference I'm talking about is not about how much body fat we have, or where it ends up. I'm talking about the chemical nature of our body fat.

As you read in the introduction, we consume a lot of vegetable oils these days. Most people are not sure what vegetable oils are or where they come from. People often assume vegetable oil comes from junk foods and if they don't eat junk foods they don't have to think about it. That's exactly what those who sell you vegetable oil want you to believe. If you're health-conscious, then vegetable oil still gets into your body by way of foods that manufacturers work hard to convince you are healthy. A shocking 80 percent of the average American's fat calories come from vegetable oils, leaving very little room for the healthy fats your cells actually crave. Most of the vegetable oil in your body right now does not come from cooking oils you purposefully added—instead, most of it comes from restaurant meals and packaged foods you've eaten.

The fatty acids in these vegetable oils must be stored in your body fat, as your body has no way of eliminating them. Over time, as you continue to eat more and more vegetable oils, the fatty acid composition of your body fat changes. Instead of reflecting the fatty acid profile nature has created to suit our energy needs, the fatty acid composition increasingly reflects the composition of the vegetable oils. Unlike the fatty acids in foods we should be eating, the fatty acids in vegetable oils are difficult for your body to burn in a controlled fashion, and cells can't extract energy from them with normal efficiency (we'll go into this in more detail in Part Two later on).

Your body fat is supposed to be your primary cellular fuel. When you can't burn your body fat for energy, your cells are forced to turn to the less reliable alternative fuel: sugar. In later chapters we are going to discuss the powerful impact of those vegetable-oil-derived fatty acids on energy and metabolism. What I want to do right now is introduce you to the energy challenges faced when your body is forced to rely more heavily on sugar.

Sugar is a less reliable fuel than body fat due to the simple physiologic reality that our body can neither store it in adequate quantities nor transport it through the bloodstream in adequate amounts. For reasons we'll soon discover, an unreliable fuel supply means your cellular engines will sometimes fail to fire on all cylinders.

Trying to live life while your cellular engines are not firing on all cylinders is going to force you to make compromises. It's a little like trying to run a fleet of delivery trucks with unreliable engines that constantly stall or slow your vehicles down, delaying deliveries by hours or days at a time. Obviously, your business is not going to thrive the way it would given a fleet of fully operational vehicles. Right now, with blocked fatburn, your body is unable to thrive the way it would given a steady supply of energy.

BURNING BODY FAT PROMOTES WEIGHT LOSS. BURNING SUGAR DOES NOT.

Aside from the energy advantages of burning body fat, burning body fat makes losing weight much easier. The advantage comes in large part from the simple and undeniable fact that when you want to lose weight, you want to get rid of your excess body fat, which is by definition made of body fat. Not sugar.

Even though this argument may seem obvious, when you visit a typical dietitian or read the typical weight loss literature, all the focus is on sugar. You don't hear much at all about what to do specifically to burn off your body fat. You're told to eat fruit, which is loaded with sugar, or whole grains like oatmeal, which your digestive system breaks down into almost nothing but sugar. You're told to eat frequently, in small amounts, to keep you from feeling hungry, or cranky, by keeping your blood sugar up. You're also typically told that you need to exercise to lose weight—and here's where you might think you'll burn fat. But wherever you go to exercise, the trainers typically tell you that for lifting weights or exercising at high intensity, you need to support muscle glycogen by fueling up with sports beverages or other products that are typically sweetened with sugar.

Let's talk a moment about where sugar comes from, because even when they don't specifically mention sugar, when dietitians or anyone else advise eating fruits, pasta, and breads made with flours—including whole grain flours—or starchy foods like potatoes and rice, they're still telling you to eat foods that will raise your blood sugar. Why do fruits and pasta and so on raise your sugar? Because fruits and starches are loaded with sugar. Your digestive system breaks down fruit to extract the natural sugars. It also breaks down starches from flours, rice, and potatoes into sugar. What about whole grain flour, brown rice, and sweet potatoes? Those all get rapidly broken down into sugar. And not in trivial amounts. An apple, for instance, has more sugar than a Hershey's chocolate bar; so do two small slices of bread. Even though fruit sugar is totally natural and unrefined, sugar is sugar. And once sugar gets in your bloodstream, it has the same harmful effects whether it came from oatmeal, orange slices, or Oreos. In other words, well-meaning people are unfortunately advising you to eat foods that are likely to raise your blood sugar, which is ultimately harmful to your health.

Burning body fat for fuel not only energizes you in ways that support weight loss; it also gives you a huge collection of tangible health advantages not available to you while your cells are dependent on sugar because burning body fat enables your cells to produce a special kind of brain fuel, called ketones. These advantages were largely unknown until very recently (we'll learn more about ketones in Part Two).

YOUR BODY IS DESIGNED TO BURN MOSTLY FAT, NOT SUGAR

Many health professionals still believe that if you don't have any weight to lose, the sort of fuel you're burning makes zero difference to your health.

But burning body fat gives us all kinds of health advantages. Some have to do with ketones, and some have to do with the simple fact that body fat provides you with a steady supply of energy.

Here are five basic but underappreciated facts of physiology that explain why your body will become far more energized as you train your metabolism for burning body fat and lose your dependence on sugar.

1. Our bloodstream can't carry much sugar at any one time, so sugar burners suffer from frequent energy deficits. At a normal blood sugar level, our bloodstream contains only 4 grams, which translates to about 16 calories. Much more than that damages your tissues because sugar is so sticky that it sticks to all your body tissues, glomming them up. Fat, on the other hand, is not sticky, so it does not glom up your body tissues. If you are a good fatburner, then the amount of cellular energy available in your bloodstream at rest equates to about 60 calories. During exercise, a healthy metabolism can easily dump ten times that amount of calories into your bloodstream. Having more calories in your bloodstream means your body is literally pulsing with energy.

2. We don't have a lot of space to store sugar in our body, and only the liver can release its stored sugar back into the bloodstream. The average liver stores less than 50 or so grams of sugar as glycogen, and women tend to store even less. 50 grams represents 200 calories. Most people burn about 1 to 2 calories per minute at rest and 2 to 3 during light work activity, so 200 calories will last at most about three hours at a desk job and less than that with employment that requires any kind of activity. Fat stores, on the other hand, are capable of fueling us for days of sustained energy, or weeks at a time at rest and even longer if we're overweight.

3. If you eat more than a few grams of sugar when your glycogen stores are full, this forces your body to convert the extra into fat. Eating fruit, bread, chips or starchy snacks, and other high-carbohydrate foods multiple times a day forces our hormones into fat-building mode every time. Once we're in fat-building mode, it's

going to be several hours before we can start releasing body fat from storage again. Eating fat, on the other hand, does not have the same effect on our hormones. Once we've burned off or stored any fat from a recent meal, we can get about the business of releasing it back into the bloodstream much more quickly, thus giving our cells a shot at burning it.

4. Foods that raise our blood sugar don't trigger a sense of fullness. That makes sweets and starches very easy to overeat, and overeating makes us tired. When you eat foods with fat, they make you feel full. So when you avoid blood-sugar-elevating foods, you are less likely to overeat than when you don't. This is why my patients who can consistently avoid sweet and starchy foods can start being more active and more productive at work even in the early phases of the plan.

5. Sweet-tasting foods intensify your desire for more sweet-tasting foods, creating sugar addiction. Sweet-food addictions, as with all substance addictions, will so powerfully disrupt the mood and reward system in your brain that you start to depend on sweet flavors for your sense of well-being. When your brain depends on sweet tastes and the rush of blood sugar that follows sweet taste for you to feel good, you start to believe that you need sugar to feel good. Rather than creating any kind of desire to be active, say, after work, your brain creates a desire to rest and eat. Once your brain stops convincing you that you need sugar to feel good, you will find yourself more able to get that same good feeling from other life activities, which is essential to helping you enjoy some regular exercise.

Clearly, even though we often equate sugar with energy, the human body is not designed to get energy from sugar. Our bodies are designed for a fat-based energy economy, and that's why we store extra dietary sugar as body fat.

The last two of the five basic physiologic facts I just introduced are deserving of further discussion, and I will expand on them next. If giving in to your cravings has fostered a negative self-image, what you're about to learn might wipe away the guilt.

SCIENCE BOX: CALCULATING THE ENERGY IN A FATBURNER'S BLOODSTREAM

The 60-calorie figure is based on the following: A blood level of free fatty acids of approximately 20 mg/dl, which translates to 1 gram per 5 liters (total blood volume in an average man), or 9 calories—plus a blood level of triglycerides of 110 mg/dl, which translates to 5.5 grams per 5 liters, or about 50 calories; 9 plus 50 is 59, which I rounded up to 60. (Keep in mind that the normal range of triglyceride levels is 70 to 150 mg/dl.) And when we exercise, the amount of fat in our bloodstream can climb ten times higher, which would provide an additional 90 calories for a total of 145.

HOW SUGAR DEPENDENCE FORCES YOU TO OVEREAT

Sugar was never intended to be a principal fuel source for our body, and the impact of forcing your metabolism to rely more heavily on sugar than nature ever intended is profound. A sugar-based energy economy is bad for all of our organs, but the negative impact on our brain cells is probably the most profound.

You may think poorly of yourself if you know you are likely to give in to temptations like a plate of cupcakes in the office or the extra squirt of caramel syrup in your macchiato. But that's not really you. Fueling with sugar has turned you into a person who thinks of sugar often and gives in to temptations more often than you'd like. I can tell you from personal experience that is not who you really are.

I used to live for my daily sugar infusion. I'd be writing notes on a patient and thoughts of the chocolate bar I packed with my lunch would pop into my head, intruding on my concentration. I used to run ten miles so I could sit down on my red bean bag chair and finish off a pound of peanut M&M's. I used to drink coffee with the equivalent of a quarter of a cup of sugar, and when that was gone, my first thought was *Only twenty-three hours and ten minutes until I get my next hit.* Now that I have transformed my metabolism from sugar dependence to fatburning energy independence,

I'm simply not hungry all day and I have zero desire to eat. I am no longer tempted by the batch of cookies in the break room. Now, a perfectly delightful dessert is a few slices of Gruyère cheese melted on dark German rye—it's seriously every bit as pleasing as cheesecake used to be. But I'm not basing this promise to you on my personal experience alone; the science backs it up.

Your brain controls your food cravings. When your body fat stops serving your brain as an energy source, the brain is pretty smart; it very quickly learns to instruct you to seek out sugar. Your brain also controls your moods and how you will behave at work, at home, driving your car, and everywhere else. This means a sugar-dependent brain can hijack any and all of your habits to serve its need for energy.

A sugar-dependent brain will drive specific food cravings. It will rewire your emotional reward system, the dopamine pathways in the ventral tegmental area of your brain, so that food becomes your primary source of joy when you've had a bad day—a source of joy that might be more reliable than anything else in today's depersonalizing environment. A sugar-dependent brain is very much like a heroin addict's brain, and the drive to acquire sugar can potentially be prioritized higher than all other activities, disrupting friendships, activities, and career achievements. Sugar reward-seeking can even disrupt simple day-to-day activities like keeping house and making dinner. When this starts to happen, most people feel terrible about themselves and are often diagnosed as depressed.

Once your brain has "learned" that body fat does not provide it with energy and sugar does, curbing your cravings is no longer possible with willpower alone, any more than it would be possible to will yourself to "unsee" letters in these black squiggles of ink on the page. The only way to control your sugar craving is to prove to your brain that it can get energy from something other than sugar. And the only way to do that is to repair your body's ability to fuel itself with energy from your body fat.

Right now, stuck in a body that can't guarantee your brain a steady supply of energy, you're living with a metabolic handicap. Once you repair your fatburn and restore energy to your brain, you will be vastly more able to achieve your potential. Abundant brain energy is the key to being the true active, resilient, and incredible person you really are.

In other words, good mental health depends on being good at burning your body fat.

That means the moment you start to fuel your body and mind with energy from your body fat, you've started down a path that takes you where weight loss alone never could: toward greater joy in every facet of your daily life. While right now you may believe weight loss is the only thing that can really make you happy, and I promise that you will lose weight, I also promise you may find yourself a long way down that road without being required to lose a single pound.

I hope I've convinced you by now that the key to weight loss success is not more willpower, but rather more energy. If we can give you more energy, we can give you everything you need to start living a better life.

In the next chapter, we'll explore how powerfully our metabolic health impacts our thinking by exploring the mind-body connection from the opposite direction, putting body before mind. This exploration will help you to become more aware of how your day-to-day experiences are affected by your metabolic health and the ability—or lack of ability—to use your body fat for fuel.

2

The Hunger Games

IN THIS CHAPTER YOU'LL LEARN

- Healthy hunger is energizing, a quest for nutrition.
- Unhealthy hunger is fatiguing, a desperate need for energy.
- Restoring your fatburn transforms your hunger and creates a healthier relationship with food.

Let's play a game. We're going to imagine you're you, a long-ago you. I want to recapture a feeling from your childhood. We're going to focus on remembering how you felt when you were hungry.

I want you to think of an afternoon when you played through lunch without eating or snacking, and then, an hour or so before your usual dinner, suddenly felt hungry, so you asked your mom (or whoever was in charge of feeding you) for something to eat. On this occasion, your caregiver didn't offer you anything. Instead, he or she told you, "If you eat now, you'll spoil your appetite for dinner." Maybe you moped about that for a minute, but it wasn't long until you totally forgot about feeling hungry and immersed yourself in a new game or new project. Even though you were cut off from all external calorie sources, you nevertheless had plenty of energy the rest of the afternoon. (You get extra points if you also remember that when you finally did sit down to eat, the food tasted especially good.)

Most of my patients recall their childhood hunger experience as something temporary, a minor nuisance quickly melted away with simple distractions. Their hunger did not control their mood or energy level; they controlled their hunger, pushing it aside and remaining fully able to function—play a game, read a book, finish their homework, or otherwise focus on whatever new task came up.

That's how hunger is supposed to be when you're a kid. If food is unavailable when you're hungry, that just shouldn't be a big deal. Children who are well nourished and healthy can play through lunch and, when their hunger pops up a few hours later, be able to push it back down if they're not permitted to eat and dive right back into playing games, doing homework, finishing chores, and so on.

So now, let's think about the present. Consider whether your hunger experience as an adult is any different from what it used to be when you were little. By "different," I mean are there additional feelings with your hunger that you didn't used to have? If you get hungry mid-morning because you were forced to run out the door without breakfast in your belly, how did you feel when the hunger kicked in? Were you sleepy? Irritable? Depressed? What happens to you in the afternoon when you didn't get to eat lunch? Do you start thinking about food? Can you concentrate on your job? Do you get a headache? And what happens at dinnertime after one of those days without lunch or any snacks or caloric beverages or energy drinks? Do you still have the concentration you need to pull a meal together?

HEALTHY VERSUS UNHEALTHY HUNGER

Believe it or not, your experience of hunger as an adult should be brief and self-limited, just as it was in childhood. Adults should be able to knock back their hunger, knuckle down, and finish their work—even if it takes hours—and all the while remain focused and levelheaded.

But most of us can't do that. Most of us don't have control over our hunger—our hunger has control over us. Not only are most of my adult patients unable to skip meals, many tell me they depend on snacks to sustain their energy between meals.

When I ask these patients how they feel when they're hungry but don't get to eat, the vast majority relate some sense of desperation. They tell me they can't function at their peak. They get brain fog or feel drowsy or even nauseated and dizzy. And their coworkers or family members may notice a change in mood as well; they'll get noticeably cranky—kind of like a child who doesn't get to sleep at their usual nap time.

It's become so commonplace for adults to regress to a childlike state of irritability when they don't get to eat at their usual mealtimes that we have a new word to describe it: "hangry" (an amalgam of "hungry" and "angry"). We are in the midst of an epidemic of intolerance to going without food for more than a few hours.

The magnitude of the hangry epidemic was first evidenced during the 2010 Super Bowl. A halftime commercial comically depicted candy bars as performance-enhancing nourishment. It went like this: Eighty-nine-year-old comic actress Betty White is playing a game of pickup football with a bunch of fit twenty-something athletes. Betty is slow, cranky, and easy to take down. Thankfully, a young female friend on the sidelines rushes into the field to hand over a Snickers bar. After just one bite, the little old lady is transformed into a tall, muscular, muddy-uniformed stud. The punchline of the commercial is "You're not you when you're hungry."

That is a surprisingly perceptive health claim. Because if you relate to the idea that your mood, ability to concentrate, attitude, energy level, and so on are transformed with a bite of a candy bar, then you are not, physiologically speaking, the person you're supposed to be.

In spite of what the snack food industry wants you to believe, improving performance with sweets—or any blood-sugar-elevating food—is not a good long-term solution.

This may shock you, but these physical changes and dips in your performance both cognitively and emotionally do not represent hunger. They represent a severe energy deficit occurring in your body and are not a normal accompaniment to hunger. And if you've been snacking to alleviate these symptoms, you've been making the problem worse.

HUNGRY LIKE THE WOLF

Hunger is supposed to be something that both guides us to nutrition and motivates us to get up and do something that will enable us to acquire nutrition. Hunger is not supposed to be something that makes us tired. If hunger made any species of animal so tired that missing meals by a matter of hours rendered it unable to get up and find food, those windows of opportunity would slam shut, ending the individual's life. Imagine a pack of hungry wolves. Do you envision them lying around waiting for large slabs of meat to appear in their midst? Or do you see them tirelessly tracking fresh prey, relentlessly on the move for hours—or, if need be, for days?

If hunger made a species tired, then within a very short time the entire species would cease to exist.

Why should healthy hunger be easily suppressed by distractions? Because your biology is geared toward doing something about hunger. Shortly after a meal, while your stomach is full, most of us feel tired. This is partly because blood flow is diverted away from your brain and to your digestive system, and partly due to chemicals that go to your brain and support a sense of fullness and restfulness. Hours later, once your stomach is empty and the digestive system requires less of your body's blood supply, your neurochemical balance shifts, the restfulness dissipates, and your mental focus comes back on line. This is one way your body starts preparing you to go seek out more food; it's preparing you for the physical work involved in hunting and gathering or farming and cooking. To motivate us to do all that work, our brain is equipped with an arsenal of feel-good chemicals associated with goal-oriented behavior, including dopamine, norepinephrine, serotonin, and many more. In other words, *hunger is supposed to be a high-energy state, not a low-energy state.* Obviously, this does not apply forever, but it does appear that food abstinence supports an energized state of body and mind, thus enabling us to work hard, when necessary, to acquire the nutrition we need.

We're going to find out more about how healthy hunger energizes us in Part Two of the book. Right now, I want to help you understand a few key things about *un*healthy hunger:

1. The eleven warning signs to identify unhealthy hunger.
2. Unhealthy hunger leads to unhealthy habits.
3. Snacking to treat it will make the problem worse. You need to eat meals that *prevent* this kind of hunger instead.

RECOGNIZING UNHEALTHY HUNGER

When you feel bad after going just a few more hours longer than usual between feedings, that is a red flag indicating metabolic damage. That feeling is not a need for nutrition. It is not healthy hunger. It is an energy crisis. And most people have learned to treat that energy crisis with something that will raise their blood sugar.

Nine out of ten adults in my practice no longer experience hunger the way nature intended. They experience an unhealthy hunger, a result of altered brain function that occurs when an area of the brain is not able to support its needs for energy. The energy dip causes either cognitive dysfunction or emotional dysfunction or both. Energy dips may also affect the part of their nervous system that regulates heart rate, blood pressure, digestive function, and body temperature, causing palpitations, blood pressure changes, nausea, and sweats.

You may not have noticed the point in time where your metabolism first crossed over the threshold from functioning normally to experiencing energy emergencies. If you've been dealing with the symptoms long enough, you may have become numb to them, and it might take a little practice and learning to help bring them to your attention.

These energy crises cause symptoms in your nervous system that I want you to learn to recognize because they indicate desperation hunger. Until you can end unhealthy hunger, you are going to be driven to make unhealthy food choices. Let's take a look at the eleven symptoms of unhealthy hunger:

1. Anxiety
2. Brain fog
3. Dizziness
4. Fatigue

5. Heart palpitations
6. Headache
7. Irritability
8. Nausea
9. Shakiness
10. Sweats
11. Weakness

I want you to look for them whenever you feel hungry. If you experience any of these symptoms when you are hungry and they intensify until you eat something and then go away after you eat, then they are occurring because of metabolic damage.

These same symptoms can occur for other reasons. That's why it's important to memorize them, and make a mental note to see if you experience them when you're hungry. If you experience them at other times and they don't get any better when you eat, then they may be occurring for another reason—and you want to bring them to your doctor's attention.

You can think of these symptoms as a warning. Just as the warning light on your car dashboard signals that your car is low in gas, these symptoms are a warning that your brain is on the verge of running out of fuel. Mind you, a person can have these symptoms for reasons other than hunger. But if you have any of these eleven symptoms between meals or when you are hungry and they go away when you eat something, that's an energy crisis and the symptoms are your body's attempt to warn you that your brain is not getting enough energy. Eating sugar might make you feel better temporarily, but don't let that trick you into thinking you need sugar to solve the problem. What you really need is to heal your metabolism so that you brain can get energy from your body fat. (Phase I of the Fatburn Fix Plan teaches you how to eat to prevent the unhealthy hunger that drives many people's need for snacks.)

The reason your brain may not be getting enough energy at any given moment in time comes from the fact that your body is overly dependent on sugar for energy. Remember, as we learned in Chapter 1, when you can't burn body fat efficiently, your requirement for sugar goes up and can exceed your body's ability to store and deliver sugar, so your cells don't get enough. Running low on sugar makes you feel like your cellular engines aren't firing on all cylinders. And that's what causes unhealthy hunger symptoms.

These feelings of energy deficiency we get when our cellular engines are not firing on all cylinders can be scary. Over the years, I've seen many people suffering from one of the eleven energy-crisis-induced hunger symptoms who had developed a snacking habit to prevent them. Doctors actually have a term for the collection of symptoms we can get when our body experiences disruptions in energy supply. It's called *hypoglycemia*.

HYPOGLYCEMIA SYMPTOMS MEAN YOU'RE NOT BURNING BODY FAT

"Hypoglycemia" is Latin for "low blood sugar." The term describes a collection of eleven symptoms that include fatigue, anxiety, nausea, dizziness, weakness, and concentration problems. Low blood sugar is currently defined as a blood sugar level under 65 mg/dl, but your blood sugar does not have to literally be less than 65 for you to suffer from those symptoms or be diagnosed with hypoglycemia. In fact, it's common for people with prediabetes and diabetes to have hypoglycemia symptoms when their blood sugar is in the 90s or low 100s or even higher.

How can you have hypoglycemia symptoms when your blood sugar level is high? Remember, the symptoms come from a dwindling cellular energy supply. So the worse you are at burning body fat, the more your body requires sugar and the higher your blood sugar level must be to meet those energy needs. In other words, blocked fatburn leads to blood sugar elevations, and hypoglycemia symptoms are a warning sign you're on track to develop diabetes.

Even though "hypoglycemia" literally means "low blood sugar," the term is more often used to describe one or more of the eleven symptoms of low energy rather than a truly low blood sugar test result.

The key point I want you to remember about hypoglycemia is this: what's really going on during a bout of hypoglycemia is *not* that your cells need more sugar, per se; it's that they need more *energy*. If they could get energy from something other than sugar, that would alleviate the symptoms too.

RESEARCH BOX: YOUR BRAIN DOES NOT NEED SUGAR

Most textbooks still state the brain is wholly dependent on sugar for all of its energy. But this is simply not true. Over the past century, scientists have discovered four different ways that a healthy metabolism can supply the brain with energy from fat:

- The brain can get energy from body fat indirectly by way of molecules the liver makes from body fat, called *ketones*.
- Specialized cells in the brain, called microglia, can also manufacture ketones.
- Dairy and coconut contain special fats, called short- and medium-chain fatty acids, that the brain can use directly.
- The colon can convert some plant fibers into short-chain fatty acids that the brain can use directly.

The most well-known of these brain fuels are the ketones. The wildly popular keto diet gets its name from the fact that its goal is to support your body's ketone production. We will be learning more about ketones in the coming chapters. The modern diet deprives your brain of every one of these fuels, thus leaving your brain with limited options to meet its energy needs. When your brain is abnormally sugar-dependent, this distorts your relationship with food, creating unhealthy cravings and contributing to emotional eating.

Many of these eleven low-energy symptoms may not seem serious on their own. If you experience a low-energy-induced headache and don't get to eat, you'll probably be fine just powering through it most of the time. But sometimes your hypoglycemia might progress and become something more serious. For example, maybe the headache is bad enough that it forces you to go lie down in a dark room and rest, very much like an empty gas tank forces you to stop driving and pull your car over to the side of the road. But unlike a car, which will fire back up again as soon as you refill the gas tank, the brain can sustain permanent damage during these temporary episodes of low fuel. A 2018 study in which brain MRIs were performed on patients with classic migraines showed that 43 percent had suffered mini strokes.[1] Compared to people with hypoglycemia, prediabetics and diabetics with the most frequent hypoglycemia more commonly develop structural brain abnormalities visible on MRI, mild cognitive deficits, and ultimately dementia.[2]

These eleven symptoms (when associated with hunger) not only indicate your brain may be at risk of serious damage; they also function as the most reliable indicator of whether or not you can burn fat adequately. In other words, the presence or absence of hypoglycemia symptoms is a better indicator of your fatburn than your fasting blood sugar number, your body composition, or anything else.

The first phase of the Fatburn Fix Plan focuses on eliminating these eleven symptoms. You will need to be familiar with all eleven symptoms so you can track your metabolic healing and determine when you are ready to progress from one phase of the plan to the next.

Now that you know how to assess whether or not you suffer from unhealthy hunger, let's discover how unhealthy hunger might make you develop unhealthy eating habits.

LOW ENERGY DRIVES DESPERATION EATING

If you experience any of the eleven low-energy symptoms with hunger, the reason you gain weight is not that you lack willpower. It's that your sense

---

1 Mohamed Negm et al., "Relation between Migraine Pattern and White Matter Hyperintensities in Brain Magnetic Resonance Imaging," *Egyptian Journal of Neurology, Psychiatry and Neurosurgery* 54, no. 1 (2018): 24–40.

2 Noriko Ogama et al., "Postprandial Hyperglycemia Is Associated With White Matter Hyperintensity and Brain Atrophy in Older Patients With Type 2 Diabetes Mellitus," *Frontiers in Aging Neuroscience* 10 (2018): 273–280; Marnix J. M. van Agtmaal et al., "Prediabetes Is Associated With Structural Brain Abnormalities: The Maastricht Study," *Diabetes Care* 41 (2018): 2535–2543.

of hunger is distorted. Distorted hunger is not genetic. It's a by-product of metabolic damage that rewires your brain, mutating your experience of hunger from an energizing quest for nutrition into a desperate and fatiguing need for fuel.

Low energy is a particular threat to your brain—an energy-hungry tissue that begins to die within seconds of a major blood flow disruption. The brain's constant need for energy is the reason why, if your sugar-addicted brain senses blood sugar levels declining, you're going to be desperate for energy. You're not going to be looking for nutritious foods. You're going to look for foods that are high in sugars and starches—which are easy to find in vending machines, gas stations, fast-food joints, and so on. At 5:30 in the evening when your blood sugar is near its lowest point for the day and you're deciding between driving all the way home to start cooking dinner or turning into the drive-through and ordering up some hot food, most folks are going to go with option two. It's not a reflection on you. It's not a sign of poor self-control. It's a reflection of less-than-adequate energy available to the organ that makes your meal decisions.

It's practically diagnostic of hypoglycemia.

I have discovered the vast majority of people who struggle with guilt over habitually making what they know to be unhealthy mealtime choices are dealing with hypoglycemia at the time of making the purchase. One or more of the eleven hypoglycemia symptoms very often precedes the decision to snack or eat meals they know are not good for them.

LOW ENERGY CAUSES EXECUTIVE DYSFUNCTION

Some people's low-energy symptoms take the form of concentration problems—which people often describe as "brain fog"—and irritable mood. These symptoms represent impairments in an aspect of cognition and thinking ability called *executive function*. Executive function skills are required for a number of tasks that we sometimes take for granted, including organizing, planning, and prioritizing, starting tasks, and staying focused on them to completion. Unfortunately, when we experience problems with staying organized, planning well, and prioritizing properly, we don't always notice it as it's happening.

Whether you recognize it or not, impaired executive function can cause extreme difficulty doing the complex planning required to make a shopping list, go shopping, plan out meals, or make meals from what you have on hand on the fly. Executive dysfunction is pretty much a guarantee that you will periodically struggle with desperation hunger that will force you to seek out fast food, junk food, comfort foods, and beverages you know are not good for you.

If you know a little about attention deficit disorders, you may be familiar with the term "executive function." Executive function is impaired in children and adults with attention deficit disorders like ADD and ADHD. Overweight and obesity are also associated with poor executive function, and doctors have observed that prescribing overweight patients medications to help with attention deficit unexpectedly reduced their tendency to engage in particularly unhealthy bouts of overeating known as *binges*.

After a binge, patients often feel so bad about themselves they give up on trying to eat well. In 2010, the FDA approved an ADD medication called lisdexamfetamine specifically for binge-eating disorder. Having used similar medications on children and adults with ADD, I was comfortable with the risks, and furthermore, I'd noticed appetite suppressants often improved people's concentration and focus, very much as ADD medications would. The two drugs are very different, but they actually both create their effects by increasing levels of the same kinds of activating brain chemicals: serotonin and dopamine. So I started to prescribe it.

The first overweight patient for whom I prescribed the ADD medication, a nurse named Jenny who worked the swing shift at a local hospital, returned a few weeks later already 12 pounds lighter. She had stopped making the spur-of-the-moment decision to turn in to a twenty-four-hour Dairy Queen on her way home after work. At first, I suspected her newfound impulse control resulted from the drug helping with an undiagnosed case of ADD. On further questioning, however, it soon became crystal clear that her attention deficits were relatively new. She'd had no symptoms in grade school, college, or nursing school. Her trouble with concentration only began after her third child, around the time she started having hypoglycemia symptoms.

The experience of listening carefully to Jenny's symptoms and reconstructing her story helped me to recognize the connection between low brain energy, hypoglycemia symptoms, and poor impulse control that I now see in nearly every one of my patients.

Since then, I've come to see a powerful connection between hypoglycemia symptoms at certain key times of the day that totally demolish a patient's ability to pull it together to make a healthy meal, which quickly leads to falling off a program. This has convinced me that eliminating hypoglycemia symptoms is absolutely essential to long-term success.

Actually, I shouldn't say *eliminating* hypoglycemia symptoms is essential for success because you might think I'm suggesting you snack on something to eliminate them. I should say *preventing* hypoglycemia symptoms instead. Preventing hypoglycemia symptoms is a superior strategy, and the first phase of the Fatburn Fix Plan helps you to quit your snacking habit by preventing hypoglycemia. It accomplishes both by providing your brain with more energy.

The path to a healthy lifestyle is paved with healthy habits, and providing your brain with energy is essential for developing those habits. Most people with weight to lose have a number of eating habits that need to change. Any change is hard, but habit change is particularly hard. Learning a new habit can be far more difficult than learning a new skill because it often requires unlearning an old habit.

Let's take a look at how hypoglycemia symptoms can create a set of snacking habits that you may not even know you've developed and that, until they are eliminated, can derail all your well-intentioned efforts.

HABITS ARE SHORTCUTS FOR YOUR MIND

Have you ever tried to show someone how to do something, like tie a knot, only to discover that if you stopped halfway through the process you couldn't finish the knot, and the only way you yourself could manage to tie the very same knot you've tied thousands of times was to start from the beginning again? This occurs because the brain can become so effective at making things easy for us that we can lose all awareness of details of commonly repeated tasks learned long ago. The part of the brain responsible for conscious motion, the motor cortex, lost all the wiring for those in-between steps of tying your shoelaces because the part of the brain responsible for unconscious motion, the cerebellum, completely took over the job, and has been tying your shoelaces for you for years without you really noticing.

Once we have developed a habit, we can do some very complex tasks without having to concentrate on what we're doing. The only downside of this autopilot feature of our brain is that sometimes we can completely forget what we did.

Has that ever happened to you? You thought you forgot to turn off the stove before leaving the house, but after driving back home to check, you discover you had already turned it off? Or maybe you meant to drive to the store on the way home from work but you accidentally drove all the way home? These slipups are not forgetfulness. They're simply by-products of mastering a series of behaviors. It turns out that once you initiate a task that has become a habit, it's so easy to complete the task that it's actually harder to stop in the middle of the task than follow it through to the end.

After years of trying to help people lose their extra weight, when I finally recognized that I needed to pay more attention to how much people are snacking, I very soon discovered that many folks with weight to lose are not aware of how much or how often they snack—making it hard for me to assess the magnitude of the issue. Snackers of all manner of snack foods have typically developed the habit without even trying. Few consciously intended for snacking to become a regular thing; most have completely lost touch with how often they snack, and some don't even realize they snack at all.

When you feel tired or weak a few hours after a meal and eating something makes you feel better, it's natural to conclude that your last meal was too low in calories to sustain you until the next. In other words, you feel like you didn't eat enough and now you need to eat more. But the fact is, your meals are not supposed to sustain your energy. What is? Your body fat! The fact that your body fat is there to sustain you between meals is one of the most powerful concepts that helps relieve folks of a mental block around snacking.

Recognizing the mental block around snacking has revolutionized how I work with people. For some folks, if snacking has become a habit, it's almost as hard to get them to recognize they're actually snacking as it is to help them stop. Of course, some folks truly don't snack but still are unaware they overeat because they get their extra calories by habitually overeating at meals. Either way, it's a metabolically driven problem and the solution is the same: we have to fix your metabolism and get you to stop. And to do that, it helps if you carefully consider the possibility you might be snacking or eating mindlessly.

One way to become conscious of how much and how often you are eating is to complete a daily food journal. Many people find that writing down everything they put in their mouths, even what they drink, wakes them up to the reality of how often they snack and how much they consume.

Habitual snacking can seem like an eating disorder, but it's a completely different animal. The difference is that eating disorders are thought to be rooted in an emotional problem while habitual snacking is very likely rooted in metabolic problems. If we fix the metabolic problem, we have hope of fixing the habitual snacking. If we don't fix the metabolic problem, we have little hope. Of course, eating disorders can also promote habitual snacking, and therapy can help, but keep in mind that fixing metabolic damage that promotes overeating will make the eating disorder much easier to treat.

LOW ENERGY CAN MAKE YOU A COUCH POTATO

Sugar dependence can also make you hate exercise, potentially even convincing you that age or hormonal changes have turned you into a couch potato. Don't let it.

One of the little-known side effects of following a calorie-restriction diet is reduced activity. Most people don't really notice the moment their body starts telling them to rest and take it easy, but nonetheless, as time passes and getting up and being active becomes more uncomfortable, you make accommodations to your body's needs. You may stop taking the stairs, opting instead for the elevator. Instead of parking in the first slot, you may find you drive around for a few minutes looking for the closest spot. Instead of having the energy you need to shop, cook, and clean up afterward, you find ways to avoid all that, turning to fast food and convenience foods instead to save you the trouble. Subconsciously limiting your activity is a common reason that diets fail; even though you've cut your calories, you've also cut your activity.

You may never have had a ton of energy. You may never have loved exercise enough to join a gym or sign up to a team. If you're sitting in your house or at your desk, chances are you're mere steps away from tempting foods. You're trapped in a lifestyle of too little activity and too much to eat. This lifestyle makes it very easy to gain weight and very difficult to lose. If this sounds like you, then chances are your metabolism has been dysfunctional for a very long time.

HYPOGLYCEMIA PLAYS TRICKS ON YOUR MIND

When we experience a boost in energy after we eat something, the natural conclusion most of us come to is that whatever we ate was good for us. And the flip side of that is the notion that eliminating energy-boosting foods would be bad for you. But there's more going on than meets the eye. Much more.

When you give your brain blood-sugar-raising foods to treat symptoms of energy crises, the appetite centers in your brain come to associate the taste of those blood-sugar-raising foods with feeling good. And this good flavor–good feeling association drives a powerful sugar addiction. The addiction is not just in your head. It's a metabolic sugar addiction, meaning your body can't easily supply itself with energy if you suddenly cut off the sugar.

Like all addictions, sugar addiction changes your behavior. You might start carrying candy in your purse or stashing juices in your car. You might start relying on sugary sports drinks or protein shakes to sustain your energy during workouts. You might consider it unthinkable, or sheer torture, for you to give up your treats: your fruit, your fruit smoothie, your pre- or post-workout shake, your dessert, the sugar in your coffee, or whatever else you use to sustain your energy.

What do you think will happen if you try to follow a diet and cut your carbs—eliminating sweets and starches—thereby leaving you extremely limited capacity to fuel your body? When your body's metabolism is sugar-addicted, it's often impossible to sustain your energy for very long when cutting carbs because, as you saw in last chapter, your body doesn't store much sugar. So it may be just a few hours, or at most a few days, of following a low-carb (or very low-calorie) diet until you run out of sugar and start to feel bad. This can trick you into believing that cutting carbs is bad for you, or your metabolic type requires more carbs than other people's. But neither is true.

Sugar addiction can also trick us into believing we eat fewer calories than we do in reality. When we run out of energy shortly after a meal, it's natural to conclude that the meal we ate previous to the bout of fatigue was too small, and to remedy our fatigue we need to eat something else. We don't believe we're overeating. We believe we need to make up for missing calories. Unfortunately, this conclusion is not correct and we are in reality overeating on a regular basis.

The point of this discussion of sugar addiction is that your metabolism has made it hard or impossible for you to change your lifestyle for the better. But don't let those negative experiences convince you that you'll never succeed. What you need is a plan that alleviates your sugar addiction while increasing your energy levels.

If you have a sweet tooth, or if you crave starchy foods, it's not really you that's craving them. It's your energy-starved brain driving an abnormal kind of desperate, overactive hunger. So please don't let cravings for sugar and starchy food convince you that you'll always feel deprived living without your favorite sweet or starchy foods.

A sugar-addicted brain deprived of energy might sometimes drive you to eat anything you can immediately get your hands on, which might include the worst kind of junk. One of my patients calls this "zombie eating," which feels like an apt way to describe it. It's a metabolic state—one you may have been in for decades—but it's not your true self. It's the metabolically damaged version of you. The real you is not a zombie or a sugarholic.

The real you will appreciate whatever good food is put in front of you. The real you will be able to wait for that healthy meal to be made, or even make it yourself.

THE SNACK TRAP

Most people who feel tired between meals or experience one of the other hypoglycemia symptoms soon discover that snacking or drinking something helps boost their energy. This bump of energy draws you into the snack trap. And because snacks are truly little treats, and even healthy snacks are like little presents we give ourselves when we feel a bit down, we're highly motivated to make snacking a regular thing.

Before you know it, you'll have arranged your home, your workplace, your purse, your car, or your desk drawers so that snacks are never too far away. This is one pathway taking you from a non-snacker to a person for whom snacking is so routine it's automatic. It's a short trip from automatic to invisible to the point of denial. If you don't think you snack very much, you are not alone. When you snack to treat hypoglycemia, that snack may not ever register as extra calories you really don't need, which erases guilt and makes it considerably more difficult to recall. Sometimes the only way to discover that you're stuck in a snack trap is to do a food diary.

HABIT AWARENESS IS THE FIRST STEP

Some of my patients give off a funny vibe when I explain that Phase I of the plan is to stop snacking. "I don't really snack," they might say, seemingly annoyed that I raised the issue. "Great!" I might respond, leaving it at that. We proceed to review the foods they should eat to help ensure they don't even feel a need to snack, but I know from the vibe that when they come back, it'll be like the conversation we just got done having never happened. They'll come back to me in a few days asking what they can eat as a healthy snack.

I'm telling you about these strange disappearing conversations around snacking to make a point about habit. If you have developed a habit of snacking, it might take more effort, more time, and more soul-searching than you can do while just reading these pages for you to truly comprehend how often you snack. The mind is a mysterious place where all kinds of things can be lost.

It wasn't until I read a study on overeating that I realized how seriously people were underestimating their calorie intake (and how unsympathetic people can be to folks who have trouble losing weight).

A large study in England revealed that people underestimate their calorie intake by 50 percent. Men in the study ate an average of 1000 more calories than they estimated, and women 800 more. These underreported calories amount to between 500 and 1500 calories more than they needed every single day.

How can this be? How can intelligent adults manage to eat and drink hundreds of extra calories every day without consciously knowing they're doing it?

According to the *Telegraph* reporter writing on the British story, "Experts said the delusion occurs because people do not like to 'be taken for slobs'— and ended up lying to themselves." But I don't believe they're actively being deceptive. I believe they're honestly misjudging.

Now that you've learned about habit, you know that habit makes things so easy to do you can forget whether or not you've done them.

I hope I've convinced you that the unhealthy habits you want to free yourself from are fundamentally and powerfully driven by a kind of unhealthy hunger. When you fix your metabolism, you eliminate that unhealthy hunger, which opens the door to developing new habits that will sustain your new healthy lifestyle. When you fix your metabolism, it's almost like getting a brain transplant; your extra energy will transform you into that person who is fit, lean, and in control of their choices.

I hope this chapter has given you useful insights into how powerfully your daily life experience may be influenced by whether you can burn body fat or must rely on periodic infusions of sugar to sustain your energy, concentration, and moods. If you've been reading carefully, you might suspect that a shift as profound as going from the body's preferred fuel to a far inferior fuel might have consequences other than zombielike eating and the resultant weight gain. And you'd be right. Still, you might be surprised to learn the diversity and prevalence of those additional consequences. Let's find out, in the next chapter.

HOW THE FATBURN FIX PLAN FIXES HYPOGLYCEMIA

Phase I of the plan is designed to end hypoglycemia between meals, enabling you to quit snacking.

Throughout Phase I, you will transition from sugar dependence to fatburning by increasing your cellular reliance on fat for fuel. This is very easy to do, and you will do it by including good fats in your meals. These good fats can burn cleanly, unlike the vegetable oils, and can sustain your energy for much longer than the foods you've probably been eating. You will also learn about something I call slow-digesting carbs that don't derail your diet effort the way sugars and starchy carbs do. Both clean-burning fats and slow-digesting carbs help sustain your energy because they are digested slowly and enter your bloodstream slowly.

By the time you have completed Phase I, you will no longer feel hypoglycemia and you will have started to develop new healthy habits that prevent the desire to snack.

3

The Diabetes Spectrum

IN THIS CHAPTER YOU'LL LEARN

- Diabetes does not develop because of a hormonal disorder.
- Diabetes is better described as a disorder of energy metabolism.
- The disorder begins as hypoglycemia and progresses across a spectrum.

Doctors are decades behind in their understanding of diabetes and obesity. Most doctors, including diabetes specialists, think of diabetes as a chronic and progressive disease, meaning it just keeps getting worse and worse until you die. A few of the medications doctors prescribe to treat diabetes are helpful, but the rest do little to nothing to improve your health and usually make you gain weight. The kind of diet most dietitians will teach you to follow when you have diabetes won't help you manage your diabetes at all; it will actually make your metabolic problems worse.

I wrote this chapter to help you understand that diabetes is easily prevented and reversed without medications—although sometimes certain medications are useful. My hope is that if you understand how diabetes really starts and see that fixing your fatburn is the key to preventing and reversing diabetes, this knowledge will help protect you from well-meaning but improperly trained health professionals who don't understand what diabetes really is and don't know how to treat it.

DIABETES: BASIC TERMS

You probably know diabetes has something to do with blood sugar and something to do with insulin. You probably also know that diabetics are supposed to follow a certain diet and if possible lose weight. But what is diabetes, really?

Let's start with the basics. There are two common types of diabetes associated with high blood sugar levels, called diabetes mellitus type 1 and diabetes mellitus type 2. For simplicity I'll just call them type 1 and type 2.

THE TWO TYPES OF DIABETES

There are two different types of diabetes, with entirely different causes and treatments. For the purposes of this book when I say "diabetes," I mean type 2 diabetes, not type 1 or type 1.5. The differences between type 1 and type 2 hinge on how each type develops. Type 1 diabetes is a deficit of insulin caused by a loss of function of certain cells in the pancreas. It's my belief that type 2 diabetes stems from a disruption in the cellular ability to burn body fat for fuel, which leads to hypoglycemia, then insulin resistance, then prediabetes, and finally type 2 diabetes. Type 1.5 is a condition that involves a little bit of both processes.

Type 1 usually begins in childhood and requires treatment with insulin shots multiple times a day. Insulin is a hormone that helps control blood sugar. Without insulin, a person's blood sugar levels can eventually rise high enough to cause extreme dehydration and electrolyte depletion, which can put them into a coma. Type 1 diabetics need insulin injections to prevent this from happening.

Type 2 usually begins later in life, and usually in people who have been overweight for years. When I was in medical school, I learned that type 2 was just like type 1, and needed to be treated similarly. A few years later scientists realized that type 2 diabetics produced more insulin than normal, but the insulin didn't help to control blood sugar the way it should. It was as if the hormone insulin had stopped working in the bodies of type 2 diabetics. But nobody could explain why.

I'm convinced that type 2 diabetics should not be treated with insulin— and I explain why below. Unfortunately, even though the information I will share with you in this chapter is supported by an abundance of evidence, the doctors who write medical textbooks are either unaware of or unconvinced by the evidence. So the thinking on type 2 diabetes has remained largely unchanged in half a century. In my opinion, and the opinion of others like myself who have kept up with the research, the current standard of diabetes care is tragically misguided.

The first point I want to correct about type 2 diabetes is that we've got the cause and effect backwards. Most of us have heard it's a result of being overweight. But when you understand diabetes as a spectrum that originates in blocked fatburn, it becomes clear that gaining weight does not cause diabetes. It's the other way around: the process of developing diabetes causes you to gain weight, and the process begins long before you are diagnosed with diabetes.

Type 2 diabetes is not due to insulin deficiency. The true origins of type 2 diabetes are rooted in defective energy metabolism. When your metabolism is healthy, your body is able to fuel most of your activity using your body fat stores. Over time, compounds in vegetable oils accumulate in your body fat so that it can no longer provide your body with enough energy. Gradually, your body shifts from a fat-based energy economy to a sugar-based energy economy. As you know from reading Chapter 2, relying on sugar causes energy dips and unhealthy hunger that trap you in a downward health spiral.

This downward health spiral makes diabetes an inevitable part of your future unless you fix your body fat. One of the key metabolic processes affected when you start down the path towards diabetes is the process of converting your body fat to a special kind of fuel called ketones. This chapter will explain how someone progresses from healthy to hypoglycemic to diabetic as they travel across the diabetes spectrum. And we're going to kick off our journey with a conversation about ketones.

When your metabolism is healthy, you can burn body fat. When you can burn body fat, your body can also produce a special kind of brain energy called *ketones*. Ketones are a special kind of fuel that prevents your brain from needing sugar. You don't get ketones from food; your liver makes ketones for your brain. As long as your brain can get ketones, you always have plenty of energy and you don't get hungry that often.

You may have heard that your brain requires sugar. That's simply not true. Your brain can do perfectly fine without sugar as long as it gets an alternative fuel—and ketones may be the *best* brain fuel.

If you don't know what ketones are, you're hardly alone. The keto diet gets its name from the fact that its goal is to support your body's ability to generate ketones. In spite of the diet's popularity, few people really know what ketones are. So I'll take a moment to introduce you.

KETONES: ENERGY NUGGETS FOR YOUR BRAIN

The brain is a very special organ, and the other organs work hard to keep it happy and functioning properly. The brain is always busy, day and night, during wakefulness and sleep, whether you exercise or not. This activity makes the bran an energy-hungry organ. At just 2 percent of your body mass, it demands 20 percent of all your total energy (while at rest). The brain is also very chemically sensitive, so it's walled off behind a protective barrier. The barrier is called the *blood-brain barrier*, and it filters the blood, permitting only a few select chemicals to come into direct contact with the brain. Getting fuel into your brain is no easy task; its high energy demand coupled with the low flow of potential fuels through the brain mean that supplying the brain with energy presents a challenge. While the rest of the body can easily make use of the big fatty acids stored in body fat, those big fatty acids can't easily cross the blood-brain barrier, so your brain cells can't harvest energy from those big fatty acids like every other organ can.

Fortunately, nature came up with a solution that enables the human brain to access the abundance of energy stored in our body fat. Ketones are the solution.

The liver breaks big fatty acids down and reassembles them into much smaller molecules that are designed to pass through the brain's protective barrier. You can think of the big fatty acids that are stored in your body fat as a whole chicken and ketones as bite-size chicken nuggets. Ketones are the perfect fuel for your brain, packing more than double the brain-charging power of sugar on a gram-per-gram basis.

FROM HEALTHY TO HYPOGLYCEMIC

The first organ impacted by reduced ability to burn body fat for fuel is your brain. Why the brain? Because the brain is living on the edge, energy-wise, always just seconds away from running out of oxygen and fuel. Your liver only makes ketones fast enough to sustain your brain when you can burn body fat. When you lose the ability to burn body fat, your liver can't use it for making ketones. When you can't burn your body fat or make ketones, your requirement for sugar goes up. Your body starts using more sugar, and your brain starts using more too.

Because your body can't push that much sugar through your bloodstream at once, from time to time the need for sugar in the brain outpaces how quickly your bloodstream can deliver it. Whenever the brain needs more sugar than it gets, you develop hypoglycemia symptoms.

Hypoglycemia symptoms do not occur when your brain gets plenty of ketones. When you stop being able to burn body fat, not only does your whole body require your blood to deliver relatively more sugar than it did before, but ketone production drops off too, so your brain also requires relatively more sugar than it did before. Remember, your blood is only designed to carry about 16 calories worth of sugar energy at any given time. When you lose your ability to fuel it with fat and ketones, your energy-hungry brain starts instructing your liver to pump more sugar into your blood than it's designed to carry in order to fuel its need for energy.

It's like your brain pushes an override button that enables your liver to ignore the normal blood-sugar-regulating rules of the body. Your brain needs to push this override button because your body stops burning fat (or, more accurately, your body reduces how often it burns fat) and your liver stops making ketones (or, more accurately, your liver reduces how often it makes ketones). The override effect helps to bump up your blood sugar level, which helps your brain get more sugar. Unfortunately, overriding your body's safe blood sugar operating parameters causes a new set of problems called insulin resistance.

THE DIABETES SPECTRUM

The diabetes spectrum helps us to understand that weight gain, diabetes, and all the complications of diabetes begin as a cellular energy problem.

The diabetes spectrum looks like this.

THE DIABETES SPECTRUM

Progressive Metabolic Damage

Hypoglycemia—> Insulin Resistance —> Prediabetes—> Diabetes

On the far right, we have full-blown diabetes type 2. Just preceding diabetes, to the left of diabetes on the spectrum, we see a condition called prediabetes. To the left of that, we see a condition called insulin resistance. And just to the left of that, on the leftmost side of the spectrum, we see a condition called hypoglycemia.

Hypoglycemia is the first disorder on the diabetes spectrum. If you have hypoglycemia, you are set up for progressing through the other phases. Why? Because most people treat hypoglycemia symptoms by eating larger quantities of the same foods that caused hypoglycemia to develop in the first place. Eating more accelerates the metabolic damage, which leads to the second phase of the diabetes spectrum, insulin resistance. And if you continue eating the same fatburn-blocking foods, you will over time progress through the last two phases, prediabetes and diabetes.

You don't necessarily need to have hypoglycemia symptoms before every meal to be considered hypoglycemic. You will develop the symptoms during those times that your brain is demanding more sugar than your body is delivering.

To understand how your body gets into trouble when your brain asks your liver to make more sugar than your blood is supposed to carry, let's look at how your blood sugar level is regulated. This discussion will also help to explain why most people who suffer from hypoglycemia feel like their blood sugar is low when in fact it's actually normal.

YOUR BLOOD SUGAR SET POINT IS DETERMINED BY TWO DIFFERENT ORGANS

The blood sugar set point is the blood sugar level your body aims for whenever possible. When you eat something sugary, your blood sugar rises. But as soon as your body can manage to do so, it tries to push the high levels back into the normal range.

Your fasting blood sugar is the blood sugar reading you get when you first wake up in the morning, before you eat or drink anything and before you've done any activity. Your fasting blood sugar is particularly important because it is the most accurate and reliable reflection of your current blood sugar set point.

All healthy people have the same set point. It's only when your metabolism is damaged that the set point can no longer be maintained.

Your body's set point is regulated by two organs: the pancreas and the brain. For your body to operate normally, your fasting blood sugar set point should be the same in both of the body's two most important blood-sugar-regulating organs: the pancreas and the brain. But when your fatburn declines, it's your brain that experiences energy crises, not your pancreas. Your brain wants more sugar than it's getting. And to get that sugar, your brain instructs your liver to elevate your blood sugar by releasing more, which raises your fasting blood sugar.

Raising your fasting blood sugar is the entry point to the diabetes spectrum.

I'm now going to walk you through the set of ever-increasing metabolic disturbances that ultimately cause diabetes. This process is the most important and least understood phenomenon in current medical practice. Let's take a look at how you progress from hypoglycemia to the other stages on the diabetes spectrum.

HYPOGLYCEMIA

As we've discussed, hypoglycemia represents the very beginning of the se-
quence of increasing metabolic disruptions that eventually leads to diabetes. If you have hypoglycemia, it's because your cells can't get quite enough
energy from fat to make it all the way between meals. At first, you'll only
feel symptoms of hypoglycemia just before your next meal or if you have
to eat later than usual.

I've observed that most people with hypoglycemia usually have normal
fasting blood sugar levels, even while the symptoms are occurring. This
suggests that their brain's blood sugar set point is already higher than it
should be.

Meanwhile, unaware of the brain's need for more sugar, the pancreas
tries to drive the sugar back down to where it's always been—normal range
(65–85). To do this, the pancreas releases the hormone insulin to move
sugar out of the bloodstream and into fat cells, and thus reduce your blood
sugar.

And here's where things get really problematic for your body. The extra
insulin shoving sugar into your fat cells means you start to get hungry between meals faster than you used to, and you start to build fat sooner. This
makes you start to gain weight.

The extra insulin is also a problem for your liver, which is caught in a
battle between the pancreas, which wants to keep your fasting blood sugar
where it's always been, and your brain, which needs more sugar than it
used to need. Insulin, from the pancreas, travels to the liver and tells the
liver to slow down production of sugar. But a special part of the brain
(called the ventromedial hypothalamus) connects to the liver by way of
a nerve. This nerve increases blood sugar production. The brain's direct
neuronal connection to the liver is more powerful than the pancreas's indirect hormonal connection. So the liver is forced to ignore what insulin
is telling it to do. Thus, the brain wins the battle for control over how fast
your liver makes sugar.

So you now have a situation where, whenever you're in a fasted state—
meaning you haven't eaten in a few hours (the number of hours actually
decreases as your metabolic disturbance increases)—your brain is telling
your liver to put more sugar into the bloodstream, but your pancreas is

telling your fat cells to take the sugar out of the bloodstream. In other words, your body is forced to fight against itself. The brain wants more sugar, and the pancreas wants less and releases more insulin than normal, which makes you build fat faster than normal.

This is a profound metabolic disturbance, which elevates your blood sugar on the one hand and builds fat on the other. For many people, the net effect is weight gain.

To bring this concept to life, I'd like to introduce you to a case from very early in my practice.

Meet Kate. Kate's body weight is technically normal but is about twenty pounds up from when she was a senior in high school. She exercises a lot, and after exercise she treats herself to a lot of candy. Her favorites are peanut M&M's and she's been known to polish off a pound after a particularly long workout. She starts her day with raisin bran in 1 percent milk, and has noticed her hands shake and her fingers get cold when it's time for lunch. Fortunately for her, she avoids snacking—particularly in the morning—because she doesn't like her mouth to feel dirty after brushing her teeth.

Kate has hypoglycemia, which she is well aware of, being a health practitioner. But she's not worried about it because, like most health practitioners, she has no idea there's anything serious going on. But if Kate were to get injured and be unable to exercise, or if she started snacking more or otherwise overeating, she would very likely gain weight and progress to the next disease on the diabetes spectrum: insulin resistance.

INSULIN RESISTANCE

To the right of hypoglycemia on the diabetes spectrum we see insulin resistance. If you have insulin resistance, it's because your cells can't respond properly to insulin and your body must make more to push sugar out of your bloodstream and into your cells. When you have insulin resistance, you'll feel symptoms of hypoglycemia well before your next meal and probably start carrying snacks.

Doctors often don't diagnose insulin resistance. We don't even look for it, which is unfortunate because it's an easy thing to do with a simple fasting blood insulin level performed at the same time as a glucose level. In

Chapter 6 (Fatburn System 2. Hormones That Control Blood Sugar) you'll learn about this test, called a HOMA-IR test.

Back in the 1970s, a man named Ronald Kraft performed insulin testing on nearly fourteen thousand healthy individuals. He discovered that 70 percent of people with normal fasting blood sugar levels had to produce abnormally high amounts of insulin to push sugar out of the bloodstream in order to be able to keep their blood sugar levels in that normal range. In other words, a majority of people even in the 1970s were insulin-resistant and unable to burn body fat optimally. Dr. Kraft's work is well-known in the small (but growing) community of low-carbohydrate medical doctors but tragically not well-known by the vast majority of doctors, not even those who supposedly specialize in treating type 2 diabetes.

Now that you know about the battle between your brain and your pancreas for control over your blood sugar level, we can talk about how that battle might contribute to the process of becoming insulin-resistant. After all, the brain is telling the liver to make sugar while the pancreas is telling the liver not to. The brain's direct connection to the liver gives it the upper hand, so to speak, in the argument. The brain is in essence forcing the liver to ignore, or resist, insulin's signal to reduce its sugar output and to continue pumping out more sugar than a healthy liver would under ordinary circumstances. This abnormal metabolic development might help explain the origins of insulin resistance in the liver.

Insulin resistance affects many tissues, and we'll return to that discussion later on.

Now let's meet someone from my practice with insulin resistance. Liza is a charming lady who has twenty-five pounds she just can't seem to lose. Like Kate, she also exercises but not as intensely. Her favorite workouts are hot yoga and Pilates. Her trainers have told her she needs to eat "lean and clean," so she avoids fat, and uses an organic vegetable-based protein powder in her green smoothies, which she makes every day. Her lean and clean routines keep her out of most fast-food joints, but she regularly stops at Starbucks, and a couple days a week she'll hit Jamba Juice after lunch. This routine of between-meal beverages means that she almost never feels hypoglycemia symptoms. But on days when she skips her snacks, she can feel exhausted by the time dinner rolls around.

Liza's fasting blood sugar level is 92, and her doctor told her that was perfectly normal. 92 would have been considered high a generation or so ago, but her doctor has no idea about the history of blood sugar ranges—or the work of Dr. Kraft. Had her doctor known, he would have recommended further testing to secure the diagnosis of insulin resistance. And had he run across the small (but growing) low-carb medical community, he'd also know to advise Liza that her lean and clean way of eating is depriving her of the healthy fats her body needs to supply energy between meals, which would prevent the need to stop off at Starbucks or Jamba Juice.

If Liza were to get too busy driving her kids to sports and had to stop her exercise routines, or if she started snacking on vegetable-oil-laden chips instead of Jamba Juices, she would very likely go on to develop the next condition on the diabetes spectrum, prediabetes.

INDIVIDUAL DIFFERENCES

Not everyone with blocked fatburn experiences disabling bouts of low energy and other hypoglycemia symptoms. This is because some people intuitively prevent their hypoglycemia symptoms by snacking. While snacking to prevent hypoglycemia often causes weight gain, a minority of folks can so accurately regulate their energy intake to match their energy needs that they don't gain weight—I've observed many of these folks are fanatic about exercise. Still another group of people avoid hypoglycemia symptoms because beneath their conscious awareness their liver is quietly working overtime to raise their blood sugar levels more dramatically than most people's do. These folks usually progress all the way through the diabetes spectrum to develop diabetes more quickly.

PREDIABETES

The next step on the diabetes spectrum is prediabetes. If you have prediabetes, it's because your liver is making sugar faster than before, and your body is no longer able to control your blood sugar level as well, in spite of making extra insulin. Now, your blood sugar set point is 100 or higher, which will flag an abnormal on your lab test and should catch your doctor's attention. Unfortunately, many people are never told they have prediabetes.

Prediabetes can have all the same complications as diabetes. I can't tell you how many people I've known over the years who have retinal disease, nerve damage, kidney problems, weak hearts, and all the well-known complications of diabetes, but their doctors never told them their high blood sugar was a problem. Why not? Because doctors are trained to believe that people with prediabetes are not metabolically ill, they are merely at risk of becoming metabolically ill, so until they actually progress to diabetes, their condition does not merit much discussion. But the reality is prediabetes is a serious condition that the same diet recommendations can completely reverse.

It's particularly important to diagnose prediabetes because it indicates your metabolism is perched precariously atop a particularly slippery downhill slope. Your fasting blood sugar is almost always higher than it should be, and it continually sets itself higher and higher. Remember, your fasting blood sugar is a reflection of your blood sugar set point—the amount of blood sugar your brain requires to function normally. When your fasting blood sugar and your set point are significantly higher than normal, you can develop hypoglycemia symptoms while your blood sugar level is still in the normal or even above-normal range. These symptoms can drive you to eat foods that raise your blood sugar further and further, gradually establishing an ever higher set point. As your body tries harder and harder to make sugar available for energy, this leads to an ever increasing fasting blood sugar as you march closer and closer toward diabetes.

Let's take a look at a prediabetic patient I met in clinic not long ago.

Meet Liz. Liz is a lovely mother of five in her late forties who has struggled with being overweight for decades. Now resigned to it, she nevertheless hates that most of her weight is concentrated in her belly. Liz's husband tells me she eats like a bird and can't understand why she's overweight at all. Liz's day is very busy, so she can only do a little exercise on the weekends. She's on the go and has developed a habit of planning out what she eats because she feels terrible if she skips a meal. She avoids fast food, but when she's been driving for a few hours she'll eat a Little Debbie cake or

Twinkie that she keeps in her purse to combat the headache and nausea she'll often get around noon if she has nothing to eat. She knows those foods are unhealthy, so whenever possible she'll drive home to grab a quick bite of something low-fat, like grits or oatmeal, then finish her chores and return home to make a proper lunch.

When I asked Liz to do a full twenty-four-hour recall, it turned out she actually eats quite a bit more than she realized. Part of the reason she figured she was not eating much was that she was feeling hungry so often. If Liz keeps going the way she's going, she'll likely go on to develop the last condition on the spectrum, type 2 diabetes.

DIABETES

On the far right of the diabetes spectrum is the condition we call type 2 diabetes. If you have diabetes, your pancreas has been battling your brain for control over your blood sugar for a very long time, producing more and more insulin in a hopeless war against your brain. When you develop diabetes, your blood sugar levels are high all the time, before meals, after meals, and even after exercise. At some point the pancreas gives up the fight and no longer makes enough extra insulin to come anywhere close to controlling your blood sugar level.

Now, your fasting blood sugar set point is 126 (an arbitrary choice on the part of the laboratory directors) or much higher. Many diabetic folks wake up with fasting blood sugars in the mid-200s. Unfortunately, most people with type 2 diabetes are treated as if they have type 1 diabetes, a totally different disease. For most of my career, type 2 diabetics have been given insulin or medications that increase the effect of insulin to control their blood sugars. While this practice does make their blood sugars look a little better, it actually makes some people feel significantly worse. Furthermore, in giving folks with too much insulin in their bodies more insulin, we do nothing to stop the progression of metabolic decline. They've been slowly marching towards multiple organ failure for decades, and giving insulin does nothing to stop the march. Some would say that it even accelerates it.

Fortunately, the American College of Physicians is recommending that doctors stop pushing so much insulin on people whose bodies already make too much. Their 2019 guidelines make the strong suggestion that doctors should "not have a target A1C level below 8 percent for any patient population," stating that there is no evidence of benefit to using insulin to reduce blood sugar levels below an average of 183 or so.

Let's meet our last clinic patient, Gus. Gus was eighty-one when I met him and had been a diabetic for thirty years, on insulin for ten. He had developed cancer that had spread to his lymph nodes, and came to me because he wanted to know if diet could help. I told him it might. But since insulin actually promotes cancer, the first order of business had to be getting him off insulin and the other medications for blood sugar control. Fortunately, the same diet that helps the body fight cancer also helps reverse diabetes: a high-fat ketogenic diet with intermittent fasting.

Gus was a terrifically good patient, especially considering his age. I told him what to eat, when to eat, how much activity to do, and a few other things, and he was able to make every last change to his lifestyle. Soon, he was off all his diabetic medications—prescriptions he'd been taking for decades.

Gus is still with us; there is no cancer in his lymph nodes anymore, though it is still present locally. Fortunately, he has not needed chemo or surgery. As much as this seems like a success story—and it is given today's world—the fact is had his doctor told him to follow this kind of diet thirty years ago, he probably wouldn't have developed cancer and I've no doubt he'd be feeling even better today.

BEYOND WEIGHT LOSS

Increased energy for your cells does far more than power more get-up-and-go. And providing your cells with more energy is the only way to prevent or even reverse the entire set of diseases comprising the diabetes spectrum, all of which stem from cellular energy disruptions. Many other diseases once thought to be purely genetic or otherwise beyond our control are actually well within our grasp to heal because their symptoms manifest as a result of the energy-distribution problems associated with burning sugar as the primary cellular fuel.

Energy is the core of the fatburning advantage, and when you reclaim your inborn ability to use body fat for fuel, you feel more energetic. With energy to burn, you can live a healthier, longer, easier, and better life.

And there's one more common condition I want to talk about that may affect you once you're on the diabetes spectrum: thyroid disease.

IF IT'S NOT YOUR THYROID, IT'S YOUR FATBURN

Over the years, many patients have come to me concerned that thyroid malfunction has caused their weight gain. That has only been true for a very small percentage of these patients. As with type 2 diabetes, the relationship between thyroid disease and weight gain is not well understood by the medical community. We're taught that hypothyroidism is one possible cause of obesity, and though that's technically true, it is also exceedingly rare.

The accepted relationship between thyroid disease and obesity was first questioned in 2010, during a conference where the president of the American Thyroid Association was invited to speak on the relationship between thyroid disease and obesity. During research for the talk, he told us, he discovered that the association of thyroid disease with obesity ran in the *opposite* direction from what he'd been taught. Rather than hypothyroidism causing weight gain, the process of gaining weight seems to promote thyroid disease. In other words, most people who have thyroid disease would not have developed it had they maintained a normal weight.

It's my opinion that the reason thyroid disorders are so common among folks who are overweight is that both originate from the same common soil of disrupted energy production. In other words, just as blocked fatburn causes you to gain weight, it also causes a mild form of hypothyroidism. In my experience, treating this kind of hypothyroidism with thyroid hormone does less to help weight loss than most people hope. Because so many people who want to lose weight have concerns about their thyroid, I'd like to take a little dive into the role of thyroid hormone in maintaining metabolic health.

UNDERSTANDING THYROID DISEASE

The thyroid is a gland in your neck, shaped—coincidentally—like a little bow tie. The thyroid helps regulate energy levels by releasing thyroid hormone into the bloodstream, which then travels to every last one of our cells and interacts with each cell's DNA to regulate its rate of energy usage. If your thyroid produces too little thyroid hormone, your cells will use less energy and you can become sluggish as your body performs less cellular work—for example, growth (children with hypothyroidism are small and underdeveloped). When you have too much thyroid hormone, your cells use too much energy and it's a little like you have a fever; your body temperature, heart rate, and breathing rate all increase. While folks with too much thyroid hormone in their system can lose weight, they also can develop bone loss, anxiety, heart failure, and other serious problems.

Thyroid hormone is so important, the thyroid gland has a superior officer to make sure it's doing its job properly. The pituitary gland located in your brain constantly monitors how much thyroid hormone the thyroid gland is producing. When your thyroid is not producing enough hormone, the pituitary gland forces your thyroid to make more thyroid hormone. It does this by releasing something called thyroid-stimulating hormone, TSH for short. TSH is not the same thing as thyroid hormone. TSH stimulates the thyroid gland to get to work. When the pituitary makes extra TSH, the thyroid produces extra thyroid hormone. If for some reason the thyroid gland makes too much, the pituitary pulls back on the amount of TSH, which stimulates the thyroid less, and less thyroid hormone is produced. The end goal is that a person's thyroid ends up making the right amount of hormone all the time. This is called a feedback loop.

The important thing about the way we diagnose hypothyroidism is that it's based on TSH level, not on the amount of thyroid hormone in your body. In other words, if you have a high TSH, your thyroid hormone level may be normal. Even though your thyroid hormone is normal, you will be diagnosed with hypothyroidism because of the TSH. Many people with high TSH also have low thyroid hormone levels.

What I've just described about thyroid hormone and TSH is true regardless of whether you have Hashimoto's, Graves', or another thyroid disease causing your high TSH.

Over the years I noticed that the people with high TSH and low thyroid hormone levels benefit from being prescribed thyroid hormone—they feel better and sometimes they lose weight. Meanwhile, I've also found that prescribing thyroid hormone for people with high TSH but normal thyroid hormone levels rarely benefit. Sure, their TSH goes back down to normal, but they typically don't feel much better.

Some experts have taken to suggesting that the normal ranges of TSH tests need to be lowered. But I don't think that will help. The real problem with the thyroid test is that we rely too heavily on thyroid abnormalities to point us to the cause of weight loss. It's the first and sometimes also the only metabolic cause of weight gain and fatigue that we look for.

But typical thyroid symptoms, which include fatigue, brain fog, and weakness, are exactly the same as the symptoms of blocked fatburn. Other hypothyroid symptoms include anxiety, nausea, dizziness, weakness, and concentration problems. Sound familiar? These are also hypoglycemia symptoms. It has been my experience that most people with thyroid disease who don't feel better taking their thyroid hormone prescriptions do improve as their fatburn improves.

A THYROID HORMONE CALLED T3 MAY HELP MORE THAN T4

When your doctor tests you for hypothyroidism, he usually tests TSH, which is produced by your pituitary in abnormally high amounts when you have hypothyroidism. Thyroid hormone is called T4. But the body converts T4 into a highly similar hormone called simply T3, which may be more biologically important than T4. When your doctor discovers that your TSH is high, the next test he'll do is T4. Doctors do not routinely check for T3 unless you ask. If your T4 is normal but your T3 is low, giving you T4 probably won't help as much as giving you T3.

In my experience, giving T3 to folks with low T3 helps quite a bit. It's important to realize that if you have normal TSH and T4 and low T3, you don't have thyroid disease. You have a problem with the enzymes in your body tissues that normally convert T4 to T3. With that in mind, it's worth testing T3 all by itself if you have issues with fatigue. (A complete discussion of T3 testing is beyond the scope of the book.)

A LESSON FROM MEDICAL SCHOOL

When I was in medical school, type 2 diabetes was much less common than today, and thought to be genetically based. Only when I traveled to Southwest Native American reservations did I see very much diabetes. The thinking at that time was that Native Americans were genetically selected to store fat because they'd been forced for generations to subsist on cactus pads and fibrous roots, and the tendency to store fat—referred to as a so-called "thrifty" gene—was a result of natural selection weeding out those people who couldn't build fat fast.

But now the rates of diabetes among Caucasians exceed those among Native Americans of the 1990s, revealing the wrongheadedness of the thrifty-gene hypothesis, and prompting an alternative explanation that the Native American diabetes epidemic was driven by diet.

Indeed, as overall rates of diabetes have risen, rates of diabetes among Native Americans have soared, reaching about 50 percent. Due to widespread poverty, most Native Americans living on reservations are living on inexpensive food composed of three main ingredients: vegetable oils, flours, and sugar. They do not eat a lot of butter, lard, or tallow, as those foods are more expensive and not as abundant in the stores. They don't eat much red meat for the same reason: chicken is cheaper. What we can learn from this is that a diet composed primarily of vegetable oils, flours, and sugars is a recipe for poor health. It amounts to a kind of clinical trial of the ability of these three ingredients to cause weight gain and diabetes.

This little experiment has now expanded to include the rest of the country. Our diets today are now very similar to the diets on the Native American reservation of the 1990s. You could say that we are now living in a giant clinical trial that we didn't exactly sign up for. The trial has shown definitively that you can create an epidemic of diabetes (and the entire diabetes spectrum) within a population simply by modifying their diet.

ENERGY PREVENTS CHRONIC DISEASE

You now understand that the most important aspect of your metabolism, the one that will most change your life, is the ability to burn body fat on demand.

The truth is there are so many myths around metabolism that weight loss can seem an impossible riddle and an unachievable ideal. But when you've been armed with the right information, all the mystery will fall away and the truth will be easy to see.

That's why I'd now like to introduce you to your body's four fatburn systems, all of which are damaged by the process of living on the diabetes spectrum, and all of which will begin to function better as you follow the Fatburn Fix Plan.

KETONES END SUGAR ADDICTION

Your brain is power-hungry. That's why, right now, it's addicted to sugar. By giving your brain more power than sugar is capable of providing, you will end your sugar addiction. As much as your brain loves sugar, it loves ketones even more.

Ketones are one of the most powerful forms of cellular energy. When your fatburn is fully functional and your metabolism is healthy enough to make ketones between meals, you won't experience any of the hypoglycemia or overactive hunger symptoms you learned about in this chapter. After a full day of work behind a desk, you'll want to get up and be more active. If you are usually exhausted or physically achy by the time you get home, you'll find these symptoms improve or disappear.

To truly manifest the power potential of your brain, you need to supply it with maximum-capacity fuel. When your bloodstream contains plenty of ketones, your brain has access to more than twice the caloric energy as it does when there are no ketones in your blood. Just like putting a high-energy fuel into an engine translates to better force generation, putting ketones into your bloodstream translates to more brain output.

MORE BRAIN POWER MIGHT EVEN RAISE YOUR IQ

We've all experienced that moment in time where things are going on around you and you're not quite tracking everything. It might come when you have a manual splayed out across your lap and parts scattered around you as you try to install a water-filtration system, only to realize in a moment of slight panic that none of this makes sense to you. Or you might be starting a new job, and as your supervisor is walking you through your list of responsibilities, you realize that you've already forgotten some of what she told you fifteen minutes ago. We all know this feeling. We have nightmares about this feeling—the feeling of being out of it, not quite keeping up, trapped in a mental fog that leaves you feeling naked and exposed and embarrassed.

You don't need to be the smartest person in the room, but you sure as heck don't want to be the dumbest. You want to be capable. And for that you need mental acuity.

My friend Dave Asprey, Silicon Valley entrepreneur, "biohacker," and founder of the Bulletproof Coffee empire, has taken a great interest in whether or not ketones might sharpen his mind by actually, measurably, increasing his IQ. In typical Dave Asprey fashion, he decided to conduct an experiment using himself as the subject. He first took an IQ test while following his pre-biohacker diet. Then he adopted a diet specifically engineered to help him produce a higher level of ketones. After some time on this new diet, he tested himself again. If that second test score had been only marginally higher than the first, we could write the deviation off—maybe he got better sleep, or had eaten better, or had just become more adept at taking IQ tests. But Asprey's results suggest that he had gotten quite a bit smarter as a result of adopting a ketogenic diet—fifteen IQ points higher, equal to one full standard deviation, a significant elevation in mental acuity.

I'm not suggesting that you're going to become a genius simply by burning body fat fast enough to produce lots of ketones. What I am suggesting is that by not forcing your brain cells to depend on sugar, you will provide yourself a glimpse of your own innate mental abilities in a way you may not have ever experienced before. You'll have fewer days where you don't feel yourself. Your brain loves ketones, and adopting a diet that allows your brain to receive ketones moves you closer to becoming as smart as you were meant to be.

Part Two

MEET YOUR METABOLISM

4

———

Flexible Metabolism Beats "Fast" Metabolism

IN THIS CHAPTER YOU'LL LEARN

- A healthy metabolism is flexible, not "fast."
- Your metabolism is composed of four body systems whose job is to maintain optimal body composition so you don't get too fat or too thin.
- Damage to the first body system is what sets us up for cascading damage to the rest.

THE MYTH OF THE "FAST" METABOLISM

Say you were invited to stay with your girlfriend at her summer home at Lake Champlain in Vermont. When you pull into the driveway at 2 p.m., you find her coming back from her regular three-mile run along the lake with the rescue greyhound she's rehabilitating. She's pulling out her earbuds because, as a busy pediatrician with a thriving practice, she wanted to make the most of her "downtime" by listening to continuing medical education tapes during her jog. She shows you to your room, which she painted herself in perfect Ralph Lauren colors the weekend before. She has laid out upon her grandmother's antique quilted featherbed a gift of a photo album from your visit last year. The air is rich with the spiced aromas of a curry she's been simmering on the stove since early this morning. Her husband is off in Japan meeting with the CEO of a sporting goods chain he's opening and won't be home till tomorrow, and as the perfect host, she smiles sweetly to tell you, "I love having you all to myself" as you find yourself wondering if you will last the weekend.

She might seem like she is from another planet, but in reality, she's not all that different from you. While she may enjoy economic advantages, the only difference physiologically is that her metabolism is operating on a healthier level. All four of her body's energy management systems, which we'll call the four fatburn systems, are fully functional. This means her cells are able to convert body fat into physical motion with near-ideal efficiency.

That leads us to an important point: you may be thinking that in order to burn fat, you'll need to "speed up" your metabolism. That's how we talk about it, right? When we see someone fit and trim and loaded with energy who never bothers about what they're eating, we automatically think: they must have a fast metabolism. Boom.

But "fast" metabolisms are a myth. Your friend in Vermont doesn't have a faster metabolism; she has a metabolism that operates more efficiently, able to use calories for building lean tissue like muscle and bone (and blood vessels and nerves to serve those tissues) instead of just using them to build fat. When your metabolism is healthier, you'll be able to do more of this as well. So I want you to trade in the concept of having a "fast" or "slow" metabolism for having an efficient or inefficient metabolism. If you have an *inefficient* metabolism, you'll suffer from low energy and your energy will be even worse if you go too long between meals. If you have an *efficient* metabolism, you'll have plenty of energy all the time.

Perhaps the most profound benefit of an efficient metabolism is a major mental boost.

What's going on inside the head of someone with a highly efficient metabolism is quite different from what's going on in the mind of the average person who needs to lose weight. Their concentration is not disturbed by intrusive thoughts of food. When they take a break at work, they don't need to snack to pick up their energy. In fact, they might even skip lunch, buying themselves at least a half hour to get more stuff done. Arriving home after work, they're not so desperately hungry or tired that they need to eat whatever's fastest to make and easiest to clean up. Because their brain functions are optimized, they possess the executive functioning skills that, years ago, helped to turn healthy meal planning into an effortless habit that—just as with unhealthy habits—they may not even be aware they developed.

My goal is to help you to become more like that. Because once you get your metabolism functioning properly again, you can. But right now, your metabolism is not as efficient as it needs to be for you to look and feel your best.

IT'S TIME TO MEET YOUR METABOLISM

I've already mentioned that the key marker of a healthy metabolism is the measure of your ability to convert body fat to energy. And in order for you do that, four body systems must coordinate cellular energy generation, storage, release, and the drive to eat. These four systems are:

THE FOUR FATBURN SYSTEMS

1. Your cellular energy generators, called mitochondria
2. Hormones that regulate energy storage and release
3. Your body fat
4. Your brain's appetite control center

In the last part of the book, I introduced the idea that overconsumption of vegetable oil is the root cause of the entire diabetes spectrum. The progressive breakdown of your fatburn systems pushes you further and further down the diabetes spectrum, as both vegetable oil and sugar-and-carb overconsumption gang up against your metabolism to demolish it.

We'll start with the fatburn system that breaks down first, and progress to the systems affected next.

Fatburn System 1

Your mitochondria are the simplest of the body's four fatburn systems, and the place where your metabolic breakdown first begins. Mitochondrial dysfunction is the metabolic event that puts you on the diabetes spectrum by causing a cellular preference for sugar. We'll learn what causes mitochondrial dysfunction in Chapter 5 and how the cellular preference for sugar can affect how you feel.

Fatburn System 2

The need for more sugar disrupts the hormones that regulate blood sugar, Fatburn System 2. When these hormones stop functioning optimally, you've developed insulin resistance, which, as we learned, is the second stage on the diabetes spectrum. We'll learn more about the complications of insulin resistance in Chapter 6.

Fatburn System 3

Insulin resistance disrupts your body fat, Fatburn System 3. When your body fat fails to function optimally, you've progressed to the third stage on the diabetes spectrum, the metabolic disruption called prediabetes. We'll learn more about body fat dysfunction in Chapter 7.

Fatburn System 4

Insulin resistance also causes disruptions in the brain's appetite control system. In other words, once your hormones start to malfunction (and you've reached the stage of prediabetes), not only does your body fat fail to store fat, but you also experience problems with appetite regulation. We'll learn more about the appetite control system in Chapter 8.

I realize that these four fatburn systems are not listed in textbooks along with digestive, nervous, skeletal, and other well-described body systems. But that does not mean they're not real. The science you will be exposed to here is more complete and accurate than that in many medical textbooks. The lack of this information on fatburn in textbooks reveals how little our institutes of higher learning have done to arm health professionals with the information we need to help our patients burn body fat. This leaves us poorly prepared to help people recover from the most common chronic disease we see, obesity.

WHEN IT COMES TO WEIGHT LOSS, PERMANENT BEATS FAST

Weight loss does not necessarily improve your metabolism. By allowing you to focus on weight almost exclusively as a marker for metabolic health, overlooking the central role of energy production in generating health, the medical leadership has failed you. By suggesting that rapid weight loss is the key to lasting weight loss, we're contributing to the problem.

If you just had a knee replacement yesterday and said to the surgeon, "I really want to heal quickly. In fact, in order to speed my recovery I'm willing to push myself and run a full marathon next week," any sane orthopedist would try to stop you. He'd explain that running a marathon would definitely damage your new joint and possibly mess up your knee for life. He'd probably try to encourage you to follow a medically supervised rehabilitation program, saying something like, "You may run a marathon one day. But you are not ready for that now. Use that discipline to go to physical therapy, where a trained professional will help you to push yourself in the right way at the right time in the right amount. There's a science to this. And if you follow my instructions and the therapist's, and use your willpower to rehabilitate your knee the way our science tells us is most effective, you very well may get to run your marathon. But it will take patience and time."

I bet you know where I'm going. It would be very bad medicine for a surgeon to tell you to run a marathon so your knee will heal faster, but that's essentially what we do for people who need to lose weight when we say that rapid weight loss is better than slow because it keeps you motivated. A joint needs time to recover. The same is true for your metabolism.

SCIENCE BOX: EXERCISE DOES NOT SPEED UP YOUR METABOLISM

Regular exercise will lower your pulse and blood pressure, thus *reducing* your energy needs and your calorie burning.

The amount of calories you burn is tied to the amount of energy your cells need. Your cellular need for energy, in turn, is directly related to the amount of activity going on inside each one of your cells. Thus the amount of calories you burn is tied directly to cellular activity. This is a very important concept because it helps to correct the myth that exercise helps you to lose weight faster by "speeding up" your metabolism.

When you exercise, you do burn more calories than if you don't exercise. But when the exercise stops, for the most part so does the increased caloric need. After a workout, you may burn 5 to 10 extra calories over the next twenty-four hours, but only if the exercise was intense enough to stimulate muscle growth. Other than that at best miniscule effect, there's no lingering effect of exercise on calorie burning.

5

Fatburn System I

Mitochondria: Your Cells' Energy Generators

IN THIS CHAPTER YOU'LL LEARN

- Every cell generates its own energy supply in mitochondria.
- Your ability to burn fat depends on your mitochondrial health.
- Vegetable oils prevent mitochondria from generating energy with normal efficiency.

YOU'VE BEEN FED A BIG FAT LIE

In medical school, I learned about something called our "obesogenic environment," which refers to the set of modern conveniences that allow us to sit most of the day. I also learned that the solution to the problem of obesity is to get up and get active—much more active. According to the conventional thinking around weight, in order to maintain a healthy weight we have to spend an hour or two exercising every day. Back when I offered this supposed solution to my patients, I'm sure some resented me for it. Many were working longer hours than I was and would have had to give up sleep to spend that much time exercising. Others who did exactly as I'd advised came back after developing overuse injuries, having gained still more weight.

Clearly exercising more wasn't an ideal solution. But there wasn't one that seemed better.

Eventually, I got sick of giving patients advice that I knew wasn't going to work, and I began to develop a more useful program for my patients who needed help with their weight. In order to do that, I had to unlearn almost everything I learned about nutrition.

More than anything else, the unlearning I had to do hinged on the standard teaching around fat, especially which fats are bad for our health and which are good. What I had learned, and what every health practitioner still learns, is that we need to avoid eating fat, especially saturated fat. But in doing the work to heal myself, I discovered this was wrong. Horribly wrong.

This chapter will show you what I've learned about fat, and what I believe every doctor needs to know in order to truly help their patients. The most important lesson in this chapter is that your cells produce energy most efficiently when burning certain fats, including the very fats we've been told to avoid. The flip side of that bad advice is every bit as important: the kinds of fats we're told are healthy can actually be incredibly harmful to our body's energy-generating mitochondria.

Those myths about fats are the true root cause of our obesity epidemic and the true root cause of every disease along the diabetes spectrum. I've come to understand that avoiding vegetable oils is the most important action you can take to improve your health. To understand why, we're going to learn how the various fats in our diet impact the little machines inside our cells that create almost all our body's energy. Let's start out by taking a close look at the mitochondrial process of converting food to energy.

MITOCHONDRIA CONVERT FOOD TO ENERGY

If you have had difficulty losing weight, chances are your mitochondria are in trouble. Collectively, the mitochondria in your body represent the foundational base of your metabolism upon which the other three more complex fatburn systems rest. Therefore, mitochondrial dysfunction is the root cause of fatburn disruption, which leads to the whole host of metabolic damage you may be experiencing now. Getting your mitochondria back on line, functioning normally and powering your cells at full capacity, is not only essential to weight loss; it's essential to longevity and quality of life.

At this point you may be wondering what exactly mitochondria are.

Mitochondria are tiny chambers inside your cells, which textbooks usually draw to look like baby bassinets. They serve as miniature energy generators inside every cell in your body, running every minute of every day, generating just the right amount of energy to meet the needs of your cells. Just as houses need energy in order to run their heating, cooling, cleaning, cooking, and other systems, your cells need energy to run all the other little machines inside them that make protein, make DNA, bring in nutrients, expel wastes, and so on. But while most houses draw energy off of an external power grid, your mitochondria are more like independent power generators, each one providing energy for its own cell. The more active a cell is, the more energy mitochondria generate.

When you get your household electric bill, the total amount of energy you've used is measured in units called watts. When we talk about energy that powers our cells, the unit we use most often is kilocalories, or simply calories. Calories and watts are just different units of energy, and they're actually interchangeable. Sitting here reading, you're burning about 1 calorie per minute, which over the course of an hour equates to about 1 watt. Whether those calories come from fat or sugar, they are being converted into energy inside your mitochondria. Every calorie you've ever burned in your life was burned inside your mitochondria.

Remember how I've been saying that a healthy metabolism is not faster than an unhealthy one? It's more efficient, just like an engine in a newer car is more efficient than an engine in an older car. Mitochondria are the engine in this analogy, so they're the part of the cell where the energy-production inefficiencies occur. If your mitochondria function efficiently, your cells can get all the energy they need all the time, giving them the opportunity to function at their peak. If your mitochondria don't function efficiently, then your cells can't get all the energy they need and can't always function properly.

What makes mitochondria less efficient than they should be? It turns out that just like mechanical engines, our biological engines are designed to burn a certain kind of fuel. If you provide mitochondria the fuel they're designed to burn, they work at peak efficiency. If you provide mitochondria the wrong kind of fuel, they don't. This efficiency, or lack of it, is the most important determinant of your overall health.

SCIENCE BOX: YOUR HOUSE RUNS ON ELECTRICITY. YOUR CELLS RUN ON ATP.

You need air because you need oxygen. Oxygen enables your mitochondria to harness the energy in your food. Oxygen is very reactive and must be transported through the bloodstream on specially designed molecules that keep it under control. The molecules that can carry oxygen safely through your blood contain iron, which turns red when oxidized—which is why rusty iron has a reddish color and why your blood is red.

Mitochondria use oxygen to convert ADP to ATP (*adenosine diphosphate* and *adenosine triphosphate*, respectively). You can think of ADP as a battery that needs to be recharged, and ATP as the fully charged version. ATP leaves the mitochondria after being recharged and floats around inside the cell, where any of the cellular machines, called enzymes, can snap it up and use it to do their work.

MITOCHONDRIA ARE FUEL-FLEXIBLE

Machines can run out of fuel, and when they do, they shut down. If you give them more fuel, they'll start right back up. Unlike machines, however, the body can't afford to run out of fuel.

If all of our cells ran out of fuel all at once, we'd be dead in about six seconds. Even providing IV infusions of fuel won't rev our engines back up again after they've gone too long without any energy. In order for our cells, and us, to have the best chance of making it through the lean times, our cells are outfitted to use a vastly wider choice of fuels than any machine.

Mitochondria are incredibly fuel-flexible. They can generate energy from all three macronutrients: sugars, amino acids (the building blocks of proteins), or fatty acids. These categories constitute the vast majority of molecules in our food. In other words, there's very little in our food that we can't put to use generating energy. Even molecules that our body can't use as building blocks will serve as suitable fuel for mitochondria to generate energy.

This incredible fuel flexibility is made possible because other organelles inside the cell work in cooperation with mitochondria to break all kinds of molecules down into two-carbon units, called acetyl groups. These two-carbon units are the basic fundamental fuel mitochondria use to produce energy. Molecules with more than two carbons, which is most molecules, are broken down into two and reshaped if necessary to the exact specifications of an acetyl group. So, for example, to prepare a six-carbon glucose molecule from, say, a slice of bread, a specialized group of enzymes located outside the mitochondria chops the six-carbon molecule in half to generate two three-carbon molecules in a process called glycolysis (meaning glucose splitting), and then another group of enzymes inside the mitochondria chops off one more carbon to make a two-carbon acetyl group. That two-carbon acetyl group inside the mitochondria is now ready to be burned and generate energy. To prepare a totally different molecule, say an eight-carbon fatty acid from MCT or coconut oil, another group of enzymes inside the mitochondria breaks off two-carbon units through a process called beta-oxidation, each time forming a two-carbon acetyl group identical to the acetyl groups made from glucose. To prepare amino acids for the mitochondria, a large number of enzymes work in concert to chop, bend, twist, squash, or otherwise alter the compound so it ends up being transformed into an acetyl group. These acetyl groups are the only form of fuel our mitochondria can use to generate energy.

An analogy would be that the mitochondria is like a pellet stove and the acetyl groups are like pellets. Wood, newspaper, corn cobs—any compressed biomass—all make good raw material for a pellet. In the same way, amino acids (from protein), sugars, and fatty acids all make good raw material for two-carbon acetyl groups. There are very few naturally occurring compounds that the body's enzymes can't manage to transform into an acetyl group in order to use for energy. For simplicity, I'll use the term "fuel" to describe the source material that the cell then converts into acetyl groups.

Even though the mitochondria can use a huge variety of biomolecules as fuel, thanks to experiments that have shown how a given fuel impacts energy production, we know some source materials work better than others.

THE BEST AND WORST FUELS FOR
YOUR MITOCHONDRIA

The fueling options available to your mitochondria are ultimately determined by your diet. If your diet is high in good fuel, your mitochondria work well and produce plenty of energy for you. If your diet is high in the wrong kind of fuel, your mitochondria may have difficulty keeping up with the energy demands of your cells. When your cells can't function at their peak, neither can you.

Oddly enough, there's very limited research in this area. I've dug up the best of what's available in order to understand which of the most common compounds in foods we eat appear to be best—and which appear to be worst.

This part of the chapter will compare the most common fuels: sugar, ketones, amino acids (the building blocks of protein), and fatty acids.

Keep in mind, your cells use a blend of whatever fuels may be available. The proportion of fuels available in the bloodstream will vary with diet, time of day, activity level, hormone effects, and more. Due to this natural variability, even a person with a highly sugar-dependent metabolism will generally have some cells burning fat some of the time. Nor do the best fatburners always burn only fat.

Let's start our best-fuel showdown by taking a look at sugar.

THE PROS AND CONS OF FUELING
CELLS WITH SUGAR

When your doctor checks your blood sugar, he's checking for glucose, which is the most common sugar in the bloodstream. The body can convert fructose and many other sugars into glucose.

Pros

- A small amount of glucose is always present in your bloodstream and therefore readily available to serve as fuel.
- Exercise and stress can increase the amount of sugar in the bloodstream, thanks to stress hormones cortisol and adrenaline.

Cons

- All sugar is sticky, and too much in your tissues can cause problems.
- The amount of sugar present cannot be increased very much during exercise and stress, generally not enough to serve all the body's needs, causing you to feel energy dips if you can't burn body fat.
- Consuming sugar to raise blood sugar back up again can shut off the supply of fat from your body fat.
- Glucose has six carbons, but only four can be used for energy generation. The other two are released as carbon dioxide gas.
- Carbon dioxide in high amounts can acidify your mitochondria.
- Acid in the mitochondria reduces something called the proton gradient, which means the mitochondria can't generate ATP energy as efficiently.

THE PROS AND CONS OF FUELING CELLS WITH KETONES

As we first learned in Chapter 3, ketones are small molecules our liver makes from longer fatty acids because they're too big to get through the blood-brain barrier.

Pros

- Using the same amount of oxygen, cells generate more ATP energy when burning ketones than when burning sugar.
- Brain cells given access to ketones can tolerate very low blood sugars, down to one-tenth of normal values.
- When ketones are available, the cell can get access to more fuel

than it can when relying on sugar. The transporter that takes ketones from the blood to the cell interior works more efficiently than the glucose transporter.

- Because ketones can be made from body fat, you have the ability to make them for an extended period.

Cons

- The body does not store ketones and they are not available in food, so you only have access to them when your liver is making them.
- Your liver only makes a limited amount of ketones, and only under certain conditions that rarely occur when you're metabolically unhealthy.
- While healthy folks make ketones from body fat, when you're metabolically unhealthy, the body can also make ketones from protein, which requires breaking down muscle.

RESEARCH BOX: SUGAR VERSUS KETONES

A heart burning ketones works better than a heart burning sugar. This important discovery was made in the 1990s, by researchers at the National Institutes of Health who created an elegant experiment to see which helps the heart to beat more forcefully. They connected isolated rat hearts to tiny IV lines that mimicked a blood supply and artificial lungs. Their experiments showed that ketones handily beat sugar, enabling heart muscle to pump nearly 30 percent more blood with each contraction. They speculated that this is a big enough difference that you could potentially use ketones to save a person's life by infusing them into the bloodstream during a cardiac event or trauma.

When I spoke with the lead author, Dr. Yoshihiro Kashiwaya, about whether he thought fatty acids would have the same benefits over sugar as ketones, he said that he was almost certain they would, particularly certain fatty acids. In fact, the only reason the test was run using ketones rather than fatty acids was that fatty acids would not suspend in their blood model.

If your heart beats more forcefully on ketones or (certain) fats than it does on sugar, this has profound implications for athletes. No matter your sport, be it running or CrossFit, basketball or football, if your heart is able to push more blood to your tissue, that's going to equate to you being stronger and faster with greater endurance. When you're a good fatburner, your heart will have more fats and ketones available to it the longer you go after eating something with sugar (you'll learn more about how consuming sugar shuts down fat and ketone availability in later chapters). Think about that for a second. Now consider that most athletic trainers and sports nutritionists advise you to eat or drink something before exercise to "fuel" your performance. When you eat or drink anything with sugar or protein, ketone production shuts down.

Most sports nutritionists are taught that professional athletes must "fuel up" on sugar before, during, and after games to sustain their energy levels. But I don't agree. In 2011–2016, I had the privilege of serving as nutrition consultant for the LA Lakers. Needless to say, my program was initially seen as highly controversial. Once the athletes who worked closest with me started burning fat and generating ketones, their energy improvements encouraged others to jump on board. The performance advantages of fueling with body fat and ketones were especially obvious in the fourth quarter, when everyone else was starting to lag in spite of their sugar infusions, and the fatburning players were still going strong.

THE PROS AND CONS OF FUELING CELLS WITH PROTEIN

Everything you see when you look at yourself in the mirror is made of protein. Your skin, hair, nails, and much of the rest of your body parts are all manufactured from about twenty different amino acids that form the building blocks of proteins. Unlike fat, which we store in great quantity, and even unlike sugar, which we store in lesser quantity than fat, we have almost no place to store excess protein. So when we eat more than we need, the body has to burn it off, or convert the excess to fat or sugar for storage.

Pros

- Certain cells in the small intestine may require amino acids for fuel.
- There's always an abundance of amino acids available in the bloodstream, in the form of the major blood protein called albumin. Few cells actually use albumin for energy, however, in spite of this abundance.

Cons

- As is the case with sugar and fatty acids, amino acids too must be converted to acetate to use as fuel.
- Converting amino acids to acetate is a much more difficult process because amino acids contain nitrogen, which is highly reactive and must be eliminated by the kidney and/or liver.
- A person who uses a lot of protein for fuel exposes these organs to a lot of nitrogen.
- A common complication of protein fueling is gout, a disease that occurs when crystals of uric acid form in the joints and cause pain and swelling. High levels of uric acid cause gout, and when the body has to eliminate a lot of nitrogen, uric acid levels can climb.

PROTEIN MYTHS YOU'LL HEAR IN THE GYM

The following myths are used to help sell energy drinks and protein shakes.

Myth: You need to fuel your workouts with sugar or your body will start breaking down protein.

Fact: Consuming sugar before a workout blocks fatburn.

Myth: You need to get protein into your body within thirty minutes after a workout or your muscles will start breaking down.

Fact: Exercise triggers the signal for muscle growth, and you have a window of twenty-four to forty-eight hours to consume protein before the signal fades. Unless you are a muscle-bound bodybuilder, you can easily consume more than you need, which forces your cells to convert the excess protein to fat.

Myth: Eating excess protein makes you build more muscle.

Fact: Too much of anything is too much. Eating excess protein makes you build fat, just like excess of sugar and fat.

THE HISTORIC CHANGE IN FAT CONSUMPTION

While the foods available to us in the grocery store changed in many ways over the past few generations, one of these many changes has had more impact on our health than all the others combined—and still, almost nobody is talking about it.

That one change is the removal of natural fat normally present in regular food—everything from chicken breasts (no skin) to flavored yogurt (no cream)—and the addition of vegetable oils to every conceivable processed and prepared food—everything from dried blueberries to salad dressing. Even spice mixes and infant formula. Vegetable oils now compose about 80 percent of your daily fat calories, if you eat like the average American.

Using the fear of saturated fat, Big Food has been able to drastically reduce the nutritional value of what we buy while managing to sell this wholesale theft of our nutrition as progress. Without anyone watching over our health, our farming subsidy policies dramatically changed the nature of the fats that end up in our food. Back when farms were owned by families and everyone's parents would cook their food from scratch, we all used to eat mostly natural unrefined fats from a variety of animals because that's what farmers grew and that's what everyone's parents knew how to cook. This was how things had been for thousands of years, pretty much since farming was invented at the dawn of recorded history.

Now, however, agriculture is radically altered. Today's farms are mostly monoculture, growing a single crop, and instead of getting our fats mostly from animals, we get them mostly from plants. That wouldn't be such a health problem if the North American climate was different and we could grow enough olives, avocados, and coconuts—all excellent sources of fats our body can use for energy. Unfortunately, we don't have the land to grow enough of those kinds of warm-weather-loving trees. What we can grow throughout North America are hardy annuals like corn, soy, and canola. The problem with growing so much of these crops is that we're now eating more, exposing ourselves to massive quantities of polyunsaturated fatty acids, which are very different from the fats in olives, avocados, and coconuts.

FAT: THE CONTROVERSIAL FUEL

A proper discussion of fueling with fat depends entirely on details that few medical textbooks ever go into, much less diet books for a lay audience, which is why there's been so much confusion around whether fat is "good" or "bad." So we need to do this pro and con section a little differently than the other three. I'm going to introduce you to the history of the controversy, and then take a deeper dive into the core science that's been missing from the diet debate so far.

A BIG FAT SURPRISE

If you've avoided butter and cooked with vegetable, corn, cottonseed, soy, sunflower, or safflower oil, you might have been surprised to learn that these oils are unhealthy. If you've been cooking with canola, you might be surprised to learn that canola is no better than the rest of the bunch. Canola often markets itself as the healthy oil, better than the other vegetable oils, due to its omega-3 content. But the truth is that omega-3 is part of the problem too. Later, I'm going to share with you some of the best, most indisputable science currently available on how the various kinds of fatty acids can affect our energy production and our health so you can appreciate that what I'm saying is not just something I came up with on my own. But in my experience, when something is true, we don't always need to be scientific experts to understand the concept—even a controversial concept like this. Sometimes we just need permission to trust our own common sense. I want to appeal to your inner voice, the one that you trust to determine what's right and wrong.

Take a look at the oils in junk foods. You'll notice they are the same vegetable oils that Harvard's nutrition department recommends we eat. A bag of corn chips made with canola oil is considered junk food. But Harvard tells us to go ahead and use canola oil because they say it's healthy. Isn't that a little strange?

Once you start looking at ingredient labels, you'll discover these oils are so common, they're actually difficult to avoid. Today's sky-high vegetable oil consumption means pro-inflammatory fatty acids are likely to reach a concentration in certain tissues that can cause significant inflammation.

Let's take a look at the track record. We've been cutting down our intake of animal fats and eating more soy and canola just like the government recommends, and what's the effect on our health? In spite of following this advice, more people are overweight than ever, and we have more diabetes, heart attacks, strokes, and cancer than ever—just to name a few of the most common illnesses doctors like me see and treat every day.

WHY THE NEWS ON FATS KEEPS CHANGING: REASON #1

With all the technological advances in modern medicine, the field of human nutrition has made near zero progress toward any kind of clarity, and the question of what foods are healthy continually yields different answers.

Isn't it odd that we still have no agreement about whether eggs are nature's perfect breakfast food or the main ingredient in heart attacks? And is steak truly a heart attack on a plate, or is it a great way to supply your body with vital proteins and minerals? Are beans and legumes unhealthy because they contain lectins, or are they healthy because they're high in fiber? What about the carnivore diet—is that the best for your body, or do you need to avoid animal products entirely and go vegan instead?

Why is such a basic subject as nutrition lagging so far behind?

The problem is not that nutrition is hopelessly complicated. The problem is that the science is driven by special interest groups, politics, and money. I recently was invited to provide testimony in Washington, DC, before the twelve policymakers who are responsible for writing the Dietary Guidelines for Americans, a document that sets the official parameters on what a healthy diet is supposed to be. The guidelines change every few years, and before the new edition is finalized, about eighty members of the public are given the opportunity to try to influence the rules.

The majority of the "members of the public" permitted to speak were there on behalf of one special interest group or another. I heard someone representing the snack food industry who asked that the DGA should include a recommendation specifically on "pulses"—edible seeds of plants in the legume family that include green peas, chickpeas, soybeans, peanuts, and kidney beans. I heard two participants who demanded that the DGA discourage people from consuming dairy products other than human milk and that failing to make this change is "racism" because many people of color are lactose-intolerant (oddly, they seemed unaware that most lactose-intolerant people can and do eat fermented dairy products like cheese). I heard multiple people sponsored by various organizations advocating for plant-based diets claim that recommendations to eat any meat—especially red meat or processed meats—are going to cost us billions of dollars to care for colon cancer victims. For nearly four hours, folks with diametrically opposing viewpoints provided their three minutes of testimony.

In the past, the testimonials that swayed the opinion of the members of the DGA committee were backed by the best-funded special interest groups, and I would bet money the next edition of the Dietary Guidelines for Americans will follow the same pattern. The first edition of the DGA introduced the idea that saturated fat and cholesterol will clog your arteries, and my guess is so will this one.

On the other hand, no doubt you've also seen a lot of reports that foods rich in saturated fat and cholesterol are healthy and doctors and dietitians who advise you to avoid them are wrong. The fact that information conflicts and changes may make you think that nobody has the real answer. But that's not true. The idea that saturated fat is bad for our arteries was never true and it never will be.

It seems to me there are two groups of scientists that tend to oppose each other. One group is in the business of fake news. The other, a much smaller group, is in the business of science.

One group gets money mostly from the Big Food industry and lobbies the members of the DGA committee. Big Food depends on shelf-stable re-fined ingredients, like rice and soy milk, whey protein powder, sugar, and vegetable oils. Another group gets money mostly from impartial sources and generally supports the use of whole foods made with real ingredients, like real milk, whole animal and plant proteins, and natural fats like butter and coconut oil.

Vegetable oils are central to Big Food profitability. These oils are pos-sibly the defining feature of processed food. Big Food loves vegetable oils because fats like butter and lard are too expensive and need to be kept cool, by law. Vegetable oils do not. The processed food industry would collapse overnight if vegetable oils and sugar were not available to them.

WHY THE NEWS ON FATS KEEPS CHANGING: REASON #2

The other reason fat flip-flops from friend to foe on a regular basis has to do with the fact that one of the fatty acids in our diets, called saturated fat, can be made both in a factory and by Mother Nature. Naturally occurring saturated fat comes in foods like cheese and coconut oil. These are healthy sources of saturated fat. Unnaturally occurring saturated fat comes from vegetable oils that have been hydrogenated, forming both saturated fats and abnormally shaped fats called trans fats. Hydrogenated oils are un-healthy sources of saturated fat.

Unfortunately, when you read news reports or scientific papers about the health effects of saturated fat, the authors rarely clarify which kind of saturated fat they're reporting on, and the reality is that it's usually a mix of both kinds. Some studies happen to evaluate mostly the nat-urally occurring kind, and others the unnatural kind. This is why we need that deeper dive to get a little more familiar with fatty acid terms and sources.

KNOW YOUR FATS

One more reason the good fat–bad fat discussion is so full of unresolved arguments is that it's truly a discussion about chemistry. And many of the experts leading the public discussion are not as well versed in the chemistry as they should be.

You've already heard chemical terms like "saturated" and "unsaturated" come up when you've heard discussions on fat. It's often said that butter is a saturated fat, and olive oil is a monounsaturated fat. But that's not entirely accurate. The fat in our foods actually contains a blend of different kinds of fatty acids. Butter does contain a lot of saturated fatty acid, but it also has a lot of unsaturated fatty acids as well. This may seem like a minor point, but if you want to cut through the confusion and get to know the facts about fats, these distinctions are critical.

When discussing the health effects of fat, we can't simply use the term "fat." It's not specific enough. We need to specify the fatty acid composition of the food in question. Is it high in saturated fatty acids, for example, or is it high in polyunsaturated fatty acids? Nor should we use the general term "good" or "bad" because whether a food with a given blend of fatty acids is "good" or "bad" for you depends on how your body is using the fat. We need to specify a metabolic function. Are you using fats for fuel? For building a healthy brain? Or for sending chemical messages? Fatty acids that are well suited for sending chemical messages are not well suited for use as fuel, and vice versa.

To determine which fats are best suited for fueling your mitochondria, the essential quality to evaluate is molecular *stability*. To be a good fuel, a fatty acid needs a good deal of stability. It especially needs to be able to resist reacting with oxygen. Oxygen is a very destructive molecule, and it can react in an uncontrolled, literally explosive fashion. If a fatty acid is unstable, then the attempts to extract energy typically yield very little usable energy, and a much larger proportion of damaging energy, as we'll see. Fueling with unstable fatty acids can damage the mitochondria, and fueling with unstable fats on a regular basis can damage the rest of the cell. On the other hand, if a fatty acid is stable, then it resists reacting with oxygen. When mitochondria are supplied with stable fatty acids, they react in a slow, controlled fashion that produces a much greater proportion of useful energy and much less damaging energy.

I call these stable, more energizing fatty acids the "clean-burning fats."

Let's examine each category of fatty acid one at a time, starting with the most stable.

Saturated Fat

Coconut, lard, and butter are all examples of good saturated fat sources.

The term "saturated" refers to the fact that there are no empty spaces on the molecule where another molecule could potentially react. Saturated fatty acid molecules are kind of like long dining tables with a friendly person seated at every chair. With hydrogen molecules (friendly people) sitting at every one of the chairs, there is no empty seat, and that helps to prevent unwanted guests, like oxygen, from sliding in and disrupting the happy saturated fatty acid dinner party conversation. Being saturated with hydrogen atoms makes saturated fat chemically stable and capable of resisting oxygen attacks.

Saturated fat is not only chemically stable; it's also physically stiff. The physical stability makes it very useful as a building block for our body's cell membranes. Saturated fat is stable thanks to the fact that it's chock-full of little hydrogen atoms, or "saturated" with them. These hydrogen atoms are packed between the bigger carbon molecules and stabilize the long chain of carbon atoms that might otherwise bend and sway a little bit. Think of hydrogen atoms adding stability the way mortar stabilizes a stack of bricks.

The relatively high saturated fat content of coconut oil, butter, and lard not only enables our cells to generate an abundance of clean energy; it also gives them heat stability, making these excellent cooking fats. (These foods are unrefined, which gives them a low smoke point, so you need to stir them when cooking to prevent burning.)

WARM-WEATHER PLANTS MAKE CLEAN-BURNING FUEL. COLD-WEATHER PLANTS DO NOT.

The fats in warm-weather, traditional oil-source plants like coconut, peanut, and olive are good for us because they are molecularly stable. This stability is reflected in a higher melting point, meaning they melt (go from solid to liquid) at hotter temperatures. Coconut oil is the most extreme example, being solid at room temperature and not really melting much until you get it up to body temperature. We can get energy from these stable fats without harming our bodies. (The fatty acids in butter are mostly saturated and monounsaturated, and butter also burns cleanly inside our body's cells.)

On the other hand, the polyunsaturated fatty acids in cold-climate oil seed crops like canola, corn, and soy are bad for us because they are unstable. This instability is reflected in their lower melting point, meaning they melt (go from solid to liquid) at colder temperatures. Molecularly, the unstable cold-climate seed oils disintegrate rapidly when our mitochondria burn them, which makes them a very bad fuel for our cells. We can get energy from them, but only at the risk of damaging our cells.

The low melting point benefits cold-weather plants because it helps the seeds germinate and come alive in relatively cool weather. But the low melting point is a big problem for us when we eat them in the amounts we now do because it means our mitochondria are force-fed inferior fuel that shuts down energy production and forces our cells to seek sugar to survive.

DOES SATURATED FAT CLOG ARTERIES?

The nutrition label tells you to limit your saturated fat to less than 10 percent of your total daily calories. Such extreme low intake of saturated fat is not a good idea because saturated fat makes for a wonderful fuel. Our bodies make saturated fat from carbohydrate, so even if we eat literally zero dietary saturated fat, when we eat a good amount of carbohydrate, we will have a good amount of saturated fat in our arteries. If saturated fat were really that bad for us, high-carbohydrate diets would be just as deadly as diets high in saturated fat.

Fortunately, whether the saturated fat in your bloodstream came from carbohydrate-rich food like a potato or saturated-fat-rich food like coconut, it does not put your health at risk.

The idea that saturated fat clogs arteries came from a scientist named Ancel Keys, who was unaware that fat travels through the bloodstream in special particles called lipoproteins that prevent all kinds of fats from clogging our arteries. When his error was pointed out, instead of admitting the idea was wrong, Ancel Keys stubbornly dug in his heels, insisting saturated fat was harmful for other reasons, falsifying data and hiding evidence to the contrary.

This wrongheaded scientific thinking about fat remains the accepted version of reality.

Monounsaturated Fat

Olive oil, peanut oil, and the oil from today's most revered nut, Sir Almond, are all examples of good monounsaturated fatty acid sources.

Monounsaturated fat gets its name from the fact that there is one ("mono") empty space on the molecule where another molecule could potentially react. Instead of being saturated, it's missing one set of hydrogen atoms.

Missing one set of hydrogen atoms means there is one empty seat at that long fatty acid dinner party. You might wonder if oxygen could squeeze into that seat and cause a disturbance. But fear not. It turns out that oxygen is such a big louse that he actually needs two seats, and he won't bother crashing a party with just one open spot.

If you've ever tried to store olive oil in the fridge, you've probably noticed it gets cloudy. That's because the melting point of olive oil is right around refrigerator temperature, so when chilled it starts to solidify into small chunks that give it a cloudy look. The blend of fatty acids in olive oil makes it more liquid than butter, but more solid than vegetable oils like soy, which don't cloud up in the fridge. You can think of monounsaturated fatty acids as the Goldilocks of fatty acids, neither extremely liquid nor extremely solid.

The relatively high monounsaturated fat content of olive, peanut, and almond oil gives these oils a special ability to generate energy quickly, as you'll see below. They are also relatively stable to heat, and can safely be used for cooking. Like many unrefined oils, they have a lower smoke point, so you need to stir them during cooking.

Polyunsaturated Fat

The good fat–bad fat discussion is made especially confusing—even to doctors—when we start talking about polyunsaturated fat (PUFA) because while we need some in our diet, it can make us sick if we have too much.

Polyunsaturated fatty acids are known as "essential" fatty acids because it is essential that we eat some. But the amount our bodies require is a small amount, something like 3 to 5 grams per day of each (the exact amount we need has not been well established). Today, 80 percent of the average American's fat calories come from vegetable oils, meaning we're getting on average of 50 grams of PUFA per day, or about five times what our bodies can handle.

The rest of this section is going to introduce you to the basics of why exceeding our PUFA needs by several hundred percent is such a problem for your health. To understand that, we need another brief chemistry lesson.

The term "polyunsaturated" refers to the fact that there are two or more ("poly" means "multiple") pairs of missing hydrogen atoms. This leaves two or more empty spaces on the molecule where another molecule could potentially react.

Polyunsaturated fatty acids are the most chemically flexible of fats, thus maintaining their fluid state even at low temperatures. This is why most store-bought salad dressing doesn't get cloudy or clumpy in the fridge, while your homemade olive oil dressing does.

If you're a nutrition buff, you might know that polyunsaturated fatty acids come in two major categories, omega-6 and omega-3. Our bodies use omega-6 and omega-3 to promote and control inflammation. Omega-6 tends to promote inflammatory reactions that help us fight off infections and clot our blood. And omega-3 tends to oppose those inflammatory reactions and clotting factors so they don't get out of control. Now, you might think that I'm going to be talking about the fact that too much omega-6 can tilt the chemical balance in your body in favor of inflammation. But this is just a tiny part of the problem with eating so much PUFA. The much bigger problem with excessive PUFA consumption is its instability. Because PUFAs are extremely unstable molecules, when PUFA concentrations rise above what our cells are designed to handle, they can wreak atomic havoc inside the cell. The trouble starts when oxygen reacts with polyunsaturated fatty acids. Oxygen can actually crack the molecule open at one of its double bonds, exposing bond energy that causes a major problem. The cracked-open polyunsaturated fat forms a dangerous kind of molecule called a *free radical*. Free radicals are hazardous to everything around them in much the same way that X-rays can be hazardous. When free radicals form inside your cells, it's a little like having a fire spark inside your home. It can quickly get out of control, consuming your furniture, your walls, climbing to the second floor. In the same way, when your cells are flooded with too much PUFA, oxygen reactions may start damaging your cell membranes and disrupting normal activity inside your cells at any moment.

Back when our consumption of these oils was a fraction of what it is now, the body could quickly control any oxygen-induced fires using *anti-oxidants*. Now that we are eating so much unstable fat, we are putting our body tissues at risk for out-of-control oxidation reactions. These reactions essentially burn our cell membranes at the submicroscopic level.

When your metabolism is healthy, your body is well-appointed with a huge variety of antioxidant defenses in the form of enzymes. We enjoy one of the longest lifespans in the animal kingdom in part thanks to this arsenal of oxygen-protection enzymes. Unfortunately, today's high concentration of dietary polyunsaturated fatty acids is essentially accelerating the aging process.

You might wonder if taking antioxidant supplements might help this situation. The answer is no. Not only do antioxidant supplements fail to help, they can actually promote more damage. That said, you can take vitamin and mineral supplements to fortify your body's natural arsenal of antioxidant enzymes (see Rule #5 in Chapter 11 for more information).

SCIENCE SOAPBOX: YOUR DOCTOR SHOULD KNOW

When the fatty acids we eat today have dramatically different chemical properties than the fats we'd been eating for most of human history, you'd think doctors should notice. Because polyunsaturated fatty acids promote oxidation in our body much as smoking cigarettes does, you'd think doctors should consider how eating them might shorten our lifespan.

The recent and near wholesale exchange of stable dietary fats for unstable dietary fats is the most important consideration in today's dietary discussion.

But it's not considered. It's not discussed. And it's not well understood. Therefore almost nobody currently understands its importance. That's why I am bringing this science directly to you.

TRANS FAT

Trans fat is the fourth category of fat we're going to discuss in this chapter. The trans fats I'm referring to are made in factories; they are not naturally present in food. Trans fats in most store-bought foods are made from vegetable oils like corn and soy, which are high in polyunsaturated fatty acids. The manufacturing process changes the molecular shape of the polyunsaturated fatty acid, ironing it nearly flat. This molecular change transforms a liquid oil to a solid fat that can substitute for more expensive products, like butter and coconut oil. Trans fats made in factories can change our cell membrane fluidity and damage enzymes, and other chemical by-products of the manufacturing process include a host of highly toxic by-products.

Some trans fats occur in dairy products and are actually very good for us; for example, conjugated linoleic acid has been shown to kill cancer cells. Unfortunately, the trans fat listing on the label refers to both toxic trans fats from vegetable oils and good ones from dairy. One way to find out if the trans fats on the label are good or bad is to look at the ingredients list for the word "hydrogenated." (Hydrogenation is one of the forty or so steps involved in the manufacture of toxic trans fats.)

FATS AND OILS AND FLOOR VARNISH, OH MY

FAT VERSUS OIL

If it's solid at room temp, it's called fat. If it's liquid, it's called oil.

FAT VERSUS FATTY ACID

A fatty acid is a single chain of carbon molecules from four to twenty-six carbons long. If you take three fatty acids and combine them into one molecule by attaching them to something called glycerol, that's a fat. The proper technical term for that type of fat is triglyceride. Your doctor checks your blood levels of triglyceride (fat) when he does a cholesterol test.

Cold-tolerant plants like flax and canola are high in polyunsaturated fats. Warm-weather plants like olive and peanut are high in monoun-saturated fats. Tropical plants like coconut and macadamia nut tend to be high in saturated fats.

Floor varnish and linseed oil used in oil paintings are high in polyun-saturated fatty acids. Once you remove varnish or linseed from the con-tainer and expose it to oxygen, the unstable polyunsaturated fatty acids begin to polymerize, ultimately forming a nice shiny lacquer possessing the waterproofing quality of plastic. Polymerized polyunsaturated fat is great for protecting your floors and works of art, but terrible for your mitochondria, your brain, your arteries, and every other part of your body.

THE BEST AND WORST FATTY ACIDS FOR FUELING YOUR CELLS

To test the theory that the stability of a fatty acid correlates with usefulness as a cellular fuel, and that highly unstable fatty acids make for terrible fuels, you need to design an experiment. The experiment would have to very accurately reproduce the conditions within living cells, which is more complicated than it sounds. Nevertheless, researchers in Padua, Italy, man-aged to pull it off.

In 2002, a group of Italian scientists published results of an experiment testing the ability of four different fatty acids to support mitochondrial function. They measured mitochondrial function using a special fluorescent probe that would glow a garish greenish yellow when mitochondria were functioning properly. In a sense, they literally evaluated how well each of the four fatty acids could "keep the lights on" inside our cells.

The scientists chose to study the range of stability levels, from the most stable, saturated, to the least, omega-3. They used one representative of each category of fatty acid as a stand-alone fuel.

The stablest fatty acid they used was the saturated fatty acid palmitic acid, the most common saturated fatty acid in human body fat. When fueling with this super stable fatty acid, mitochondria produced 100 percent of the energy baseline determined by other experiments.

The next most stable was the monounsaturated fatty acid oleic acid, the most abundant of all fatty acids in human body fat and the fatty acid most common in olive oil. Fueling with this monounsaturated fatty acid, mitochondria generated a brighter glow, around 115 percent of baseline.

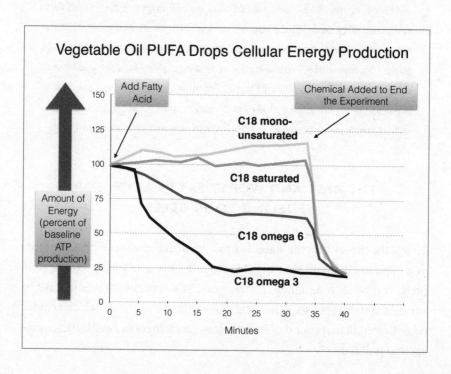

When the scientists tested an omega-6 PUFA called linoleic acid, the most common polyunsaturated fatty acid in most vegetable oils, they saw the lights dim quite a bit, as the mitochondrial ability to produce energy declined to roughly 50 percent of baseline.

And when they tested the most unstable fatty acid, an omega-3 PUFA with the confusingly similar name of linolenic acid, the most common polyunsaturated fatty acid in canola oil, they saw the lights flicker and nearly go out, as mitochondrial energy production capacity plummeted to a meager 20 percent of normal.

This research has powerful implications. For one thing, it suggests that nature designed our body fat using some of the best-performing fatty acids for energizing our cells. The most powerful fuel, the monounsaturated oleic acid, is present in the highest concentration in body fat. The second most powerful fuel, the saturated palmitic acid, is present in the second highest concentration. We'll return to this again in Chapter 7 (Fatburn System 3: Your Body Fat).

The study also raises a fascinating question: Why would a monounsaturated fatty acid outperform the more stable saturated fatty acid? The answer may have to do with the location of the double bond. Research suggests that a double bond, located exactly at the midpoint of oleic acid, may enable the cell to break this fatty acid in half.[3] That would form two saturated fatty acids of shorter length, similar to the fatty acid in MCT oil. These smaller fatty acids can enter mitochondria far faster than the longer unbroken original molecule. In other words, the cell can convert monounsaturated fatty acids into a form that both accelerates the entry of fat into mitochondria and ensures it will burn clean (in a well-controlled manner).

The crucially important discovery is that polyunsaturated fatty acids trigger a massive decline in energy production, making them useless as a cellular fuel. The study authors explain that the energy production dropped because the unstable fatty acids cause a special protein, called the *permeability transition pore*, to open, thus protecting the mitochondria

---

3 T. I. Kotkina, "Other Views of β-Oxidation of Fatty Acids in Peroxisomes, Mitochondria and Ketone Bodies," *Authors Collective* 61 (2014): 14–23.

from destroying itself. Think of a circuit breaker shutting off power to prevent your hair dryer from melting your wiring. This slowdown in energy production occurs whenever a cellular fuel burns too hot, and in doing so generates excessive oxidative stress. When energy production slows, fuel delivery slows, preventing further deliveries of the offending and dangerous polyunsaturated fuel.

Shamefully, even though knowing how different fats affect our cellular energy production is vitally important information, after this Italian study was published, there's been little other work on the topic.

Now that you know how cells trying to use PUFAs to generate energy are unwittingly subjecting themselves to harm, let's take a look at what happens to the rest of the body, to better understand how a diet high in the wrong kinds of mitochondrial fuel inevitably leads to major metabolic meltdown.

SCIENCE BOX: ANTIOXIDANT ENZYMES CONTROL OXIDATIVE STRESS

You've probably heard that certain foods are higher in antioxidants than others, and that may have made you think you need to memorize a list of antioxidant foods. The reality is that your resistance to inflammation comes not from random foods, but primarily from enzymes that zap oxygen when it gets out of control, called *antioxidant enzymes*. These are among the fastest-acting enzymes discovered, highlighting the priority nature places on preventing inflammation. Antioxidant enzymes require minerals to function and are so abundant inside and out of our mitochondria, throughout and between our cells, and in every tissue of our body that they are one of the main reasons our body requires minerals like magnesium, zinc, and iron—just to name a few.

Rule #5 of the Fatburn Fix Plan's Five Rules (see Chapter 11) will help you fight inflammation everywhere it might strike, with mineral-rich foods and mineral supplements that help you optimize your antioxidant enzyme function and prevent inflammation before it starts.

VEGETABLE OILS CAUSE INFLAMMATION

Whenever I'm invited to give a talk to an audience of health-oriented folks, the question of what foods cause inflammation invariably comes up. What I tell my audience, and what I want to tell you, is that just about everyone is suffering from the effects of a lifetime of vegetable oil consumption.

When your mitochondria are working efficiently, they power your cells with an abundance of energy while producing very little waste, which comes in the form of heat and free radicals. You can think of this as cellular smog. When your mitochondria are working less efficiently, as they are when your diet and body fat reflect the fatty acid profile of vegetable oils, they produce less energy and significantly more cellular smog. The less efficiently your mitochondria generate energy, the more heat and free radicals they will release.

The heat is one reason some people feel overly warm with minimal activity. And the smog overall is the source of a thousand health problems.

Cellular smog is released even from healthy mitochondria in the form of something called *free radical cascades*. Free radical cascades cause *oxidative stress*. The more frequently your mitochondria are forced to burn unstable PUFA fuel, the worse your mitochondria function and the more free radical cascades and oxidative stress your cells are forced to endure. As we touched on earlier, these processes are dangerous because they both contribute to inflammation.

The word "inflammation" comes from the Latin "*inflammare*," "to set on fire," and the sensations it causes in your body will depend on where the fire smolders. If you have inflammation in your joints, you feel aching and stiffness. In your gut, nausea and cramping. In your head, a headache. In the lungs, it can make you cough. Inflammation can also cause tiredness, irritability, hormonal problems, and more.

There are many factors known to promote inflammation. Infection is a big one. So are stress, lack of exercise, and smoking. But a plethora of scientific research into the effects of poorly functioning mitochondria on human health suggests that no other factor can generate the sheer volume of inflammation as dysfunctional mitochondria.[4] The fact that high PUFA concentrations promote massive mitochondrial meltdowns within minutes, combined with the fact that most of us are consuming historically extreme quantities of unstable PUFA, suggests to me that eliminating vegetable oil should be the first priority of anyone interested in improving not just their fatburn but their overall health and quality of life as well. And it suggests that anyone suffering from an inflammation-related disease would stand to benefit more from making this one dietary change than from any other. In my experience, folks who focus on eliminating vegetable oils to reduce their suffering from inflammation-related diseases—everything from allergies and asthma to heartburn, migraines, psoriasis, and many other ailments—have made dramatic and astounding recoveries.

THE SCIENTIST WHO DISCOVERED VEGETABLE OIL MAKES US LAZY

I first recognized the direct link between vegetable oil and weight gain after conversations with a very smart obesity researcher from India.

Like me, Dr. Sanjoy Ghosh had noticed that the fats people were cooking with had changed over the years. In the part of India where he was born, the upper classes had, for centuries, enjoyed an abundance of delicious food and managed to avoid obesity and diabetes, even with little to no physical labor or exercise. But in his early adulthood, he noticed upper classes suddenly getting fat, fatter than ever before according to the statistics, even though nothing changed in terms of their activity level or their access to sweets and fried foods. Lower classes in India with relatively less access to food and more need for physical activity, soon began suffering from obesity as well. According to Dr. Ghosh, the problem was that people had "used coconut oil for centuries. Then, the American Heart Association caused them to change to corn."

---

4 Maria J. López-Armada et al., "Mitochondrial Dysfunction and the Inflammatory Response," *Mitochondrion* 13, no. 2 (2013): 106–118.

He also told me his mom had been "one of the first to discard the traditional oils. She got sick with diabetes not long afterwards." Driven by this personal tragedy, Dr. Ghosh devoted his life to probing the hidden connections between corn oil and diabetes.

Ultimately, at the University of British Columbia, Dr. Ghosh designed an experiment to test his hypothesis that corn oil (and other vegetable oils) make us fat because they are poor sources of cellular energy. In this experiment, one group of mice was fed a diet high in corn oil and another high in olive oil. The mice who got the corn oil quickly stopped exercising, grew fat, and developed insulin resistance, while the mice who got olive oil behaved normally and retained insulin sensitivity. This is the first experiment to demonstrate that corn oil makes animals fatter than the same amount of olive oil. (Some suggest the effect is due to the enzyme-dependent effects of omega-6 in corn oil, but Dr. Ghosh asserts the mitochondrial effects are more powerful.)

This experiment in mice mimics in miniature the experiment we've been running on ourselves for the past several decades as the foods in the grocery store have shifted from animal-based and higher in saturated fats to vegetable oils that are higher in unsaturated fats. An excessive amount of unsaturated fats in our diets make us gain weight because when our poor cells try to burn these unstable fats for energy, the fats deteriorate inside the cell, which unleashes a host of harmful effects, including damaging the systems in your cell that generate energy. This makes us lazier than we would otherwise be.

HOW VEGETABLE OILS MAKE US SUGAR ADDICTS

If you are a normal person who can't function well when you're tired, you're going to want to do something about the fatigue you're experiencing. As we saw earlier in this chapter, cells burning vegetable oil shut down until an alternative fuel arrives. That alternative fuel is sugar. And in a world of infinite snack variety, convenience markets, and vending machines, you never have to reach too far to find a sugar-based energy boost. As you remember, sugar is a less powerful fuel for your cells than ketones and (presumably) stable fats for a number of reasons. But sugar is always around, and at least it keeps cells functional.

Trying day after day and month after month to extract energy from fat to no avail and having to rely instead on sugar may reprogram your cells to reduce their use of fat, and maximize their ability to import sugar from your bloodstream. Unfortunately, as we've learned, the body was not designed to supply sugar to all your cells all the time, and the amount of sugar in your bloodstream is limited. So when more of your cells start using more sugar, sustaining normal blood sugar levels becomes a difficult balancing act.

The second your blood sugar drops, your brain sends an urgent message to your liver to release more sugar into the bloodstream. And the second your liver sends out too much, your pancreas releases insulin, which shoves sugar into your fat cells.

In this difficult situation, it's easy to imagine you might begin to experience low blood sugar symptoms between meals on a regular basis. Hypoglycemia symptoms make you hungry and irritable at the same time, and make you metabolically driven toward sweet and starchy snacks. And as we saw in Part One, you're not going to be very discriminating when you desperately need energy—like a zombie, you'll be driven to consume whatever you can get your hands on.

Now that you've read this chapter, I hope you understand that factory-refined vegetable oils are too unstable to use for energy, and a lifetime of eating these fats can turn your mitochondria into inflammation-generating machines. The energy-sapping effect of vegetable oils causes hypoglycemia symptoms and put you on the diabetes spectrum, the downward-spiraling metabolic disaster that inevitably leads you to put on weight as you develop organ damage and additional chronic diseases. Eating natural, whole-food-based, clean-burning fats allows your mitochondria to produce ample energy, and is the escape hatch you can use to eject yourself from this metabolic trap.

The hallmark of the mitochondrial damage that represents the first stage of the diabetes spectrum is hypoglycemia. In the next chapter, you're going to learn how hypoglycemia drives cravings for sweet and starchy foods that take you from the first phase of the diabetes spectrum to the next. We're going to discover why those cravings make you eat too often and too much, pushing you further down a metabolic death spiral by disrupting Fatburn System 2, the hormones that control blood sugar.

Fatburn System 2

Hormones That Control Blood Sugar

IN THIS CHAPTER YOU'LL LEARN

- Insulin controls your blood sugar by building fat.
- Insulin also makes you hungry and tired after you eat sweets or starchy carbohydrates.
- Slow-digesting carbohydrates prevent insulin spikes, and are part of your metabolic recovery plan.

Today's low-carb craze traces back to the early 2000s, when a flurry of books refocused the public fear of fatty foods like butter and cheese and redirected our food phobia towards carbohydrates instead. Nearly two decades later, low-carb diets like LCHF, Atkins, and the keto diet are hands down the most popular diets going.

In all of these low-carb books, the main dietary villain is, as you'd guess, carbs. But if you look carefully, you'll see that when low-carb diets work, they typically also reduce vegetable oil consumption as much if not more than they reduce carbs. In my view, the vegetable oil reduction is actually more important than reducing carbs. As we've seen throughout this book, vegetable-oil-induced energy crises play a major role in making people eat more than they need and often more than they are consciously aware of. And as you just read in our discussion of Fatburn System 1, oxidative stress from vegetable oils programs your cells to start burning more and more sugar. When people eat low-carb, they typically cut out foods that contain both carbohydrate *and* vegetable oil, while at the same time adding foods rich in the more traditional, healthy fats that your mitochondria can burn for energy. This trifecta of changes, not just the reduction of carbs, enables many people to rapidly restore function to Fatburn System 2, the hormones that control blood sugar.

In spite of these benefits to going low-carb, some people don't feel well after starting a low-carb diet. Why? Some folks are so metabolically damaged by years of vegetable oil consumption that they've lost their normal ability to respond to hormones. In particular, they've lost the ability to respond to the hormone insulin and have become insulin-resistant, thus placing them in the second stage of the diabetes spectrum.

THE SWEET LIES WE LEARN ABOUT SUGAR

Leading institutions like Harvard and Yale still train dietitians to make us afraid of fat and believe our health depends on sugar.

The messaging takes many forms. There's "You need a snack between meals to keep your blood sugar up," "you need to eat frequent small meals to regulate your blood sugar," and "don't eat right before bed because you need to burn off some of that sugar before you go to sleep."

This advice is fundamentally flawed because healthy people don't need to consciously regulate their blood sugar.

Nature has spent eons developing a collection of hormones for that specific purpose, at least a dozen. If we had to manually regulate our blood sugar by manipulating our behavior ten thousand years ago as hunter-gatherers on the Serengeti, that would have been the end of the human race. It would have been a fatal oversight on the part of Mother Nature to leave the job of regulating blood sugar up to you and me. Besides, no other animal needs to contemplate their blood sugar multiple times a day to maintain a decent body composition or otherwise support good health. Why on earth should we?

WHAT'S A HEALTHY BLOOD SUGAR LEVEL?

In the 1970s, my father recalls, when he was in medical school, the official blood sugar norms were lower, between 65 and 75. Today, a normal blood sugar range is officially 75 to 99. Why the change? What most doctors don't realize is that the laboratory director who sets the official normal range at a hospital lab (or national labs like LabCorp and Quest) is at liberty to do whatever he or she thinks is best. And currently, the most common practice used to define the "normal" number is simply based on a survey of the averages. Since more than half of US adults are now insulin resistant, the US averages have shifted upward in concert with our weight. A healthy range is probably still what it was back in the 1970s. However, not many actually achieve that range, since so few of us are untouched by metabolic damage from vegetable oil. In my practice, I consider 65 to 85 to be normal—or as good as we're going to get.

Still, it's certainly true that the amount of sugar in our bloodstream at any one time needs to be tightly regulated. Sugar is sticky, as anyone who's ever tried to clean it off a toddler's face is well aware, and too much sticky sugar in our bloodstream can cause all kinds of problems. At a normal blood sugar level our bloodstream contains only 4 grams. Carrying much more than that can cause us to develop problems due to a chemical process called tissue glycation, which is a fancy way of saying sugar is sticky and it sticks to all your body tissues. (Fat, on the other hand, is not sticky, so the amount of fat in our bloodstream is not tightly regulated at all.)

The trouble with being encouraged to seek out sugar is that we end up eating too much of it, particularly too much of the refined sugars and flours that are most likely to raise blood sugar too far too fast. As you'll see, that is a recipe for weight gain. So cutting these out is a great idea.

Like anything, a great idea can be taken too far. While reducing refined sugar and flours is essential to correcting hormone dysfunction, there are many delicious and healthy unrefined carbohydrate-containing foods you can still enjoy. The first phase of the Fatburn Fix Plan helps you cut out these refined carbs, and also shows you how you can boost your metabolic recovery by using keto-diet-compatible ultra-low-carb foods from time to time. But once you get all four of your fatburn systems functional again, you will be in a position to control your intake of things like regular sugar and white flour, and enjoy foods containing them on occasion.

This section will introduce you to the difference between refined and unrefined carbohydrate-containing foods, and give you the background you will need to understand how the different foods you'll be eating can improve your hormonal health in the Fatburn Fix Plan.

But before we get into hormones, I'd like to give you some of the basic information to help you be more conversant in the language of sugar and carbohydrate and their effects on your body.

BASIC CONCEPT #1: SUGAR IS SUGAR

Weight Watchers' new Freestyle program lists fruits as foods with 0 points, meaning you can eat as many as you want. This is ridiculous.

For one thing, it gives people the impression that, because fruit contains "natural" sugar, it does not have the same kinds of effects in the body as refined sugar. That's magical thinking. Just one banana has the equivalent of more than 7 teaspoons of table sugar and 100 calories. Why should those 100 calories be free? If you also have an 8-ounce glass of orange juice with your breakfast, you've just added 6½ teaspoons of sugar and another 90 calories.

It's true that fruits do contain significantly more nutrition than table sugar. But you can get those nutrients from vegetables. Vegetables are so much more nutritious than fruits that I wish we could put vegetables before fruits whenever we talk about them. The phrase should be vegetables and fruits, not the other way around.

SWEET FOODS (THESE SPIKE INSULIN)

CANDY, COOKIES, FUDGE, ICE CREAM, PASTRIES, CAKES, MUFFINS, AND DONUTS

The most obvious high-sugar foods, these are often sweetened with cane sugar, high-fructose corn syrup, honey, and other natural and factory-made sugars. Sugar in baked goods varies by recipe, but it seems the recipes end up with similar amounts of sugar in the end: three Oreo cookies have 14 grams of sugar, and half a cup of Breyers vanilla ice cream has 14 grams of sugar, and a Twinkie has 16 grams of sugar.

APPLES, BANANAS, BLUEBERRIES, CHERRIES, DATES, GRAPES, KIWIS, MANGOS, AND PINEAPPLES

Fruits are naturally sweetened with fructose, sucrose, glucose, and other natural sugars. The amount of sugar in fruits varies widely, but in general berries and melons are lower in sugar, and dried fruits are very high in sugar. A cup of blueberries has about 15 grams of sugar, while a cup of grapes has 15, and a cup of raisins has 86 grams.

BASIC CONCEPT #2: CARBS ARE MADE OF SUGAR

While not sweet-tasting, starchy carbohydrate-rich foods like pasta, potatoes, bread, and rice are nothing more than piles of sugar as far as your body is concerned. Chemically, that's all a carbohydrate is: a daisy chain of individual sugar molecules strung together to make a longer molecule. Because it takes some time for your digestive enzymes to break starchy carbohydrates down and thus release the individual sugar molecules, it takes a little longer for those sugar molecules to get into your bloodstream.

The timing of that sugar release makes all the difference, it turns out. Refined wheat, rye, and other flours will get into your bloodstream almost as fast as table sugar. But the intact grain from which the flour is ground will take much longer. You can eat traditionally made wheat and rye breads, for example, and still get nearly all the insulin-lowering benefits of following a low-carbohydrate diet. We'll return to this idea of fast and slow blood sugar entry later in this section.

What I want you to understand here is that whether we eat food containing sugar or carbohydrate, what enters our bloodstream is sugar. That's why we talk about blood sugar levels, not blood carbohydrate levels.

REFINED FLOURS (THESE SPIKE INSULIN)

BREAD, BAGELS, ENGLISH MUFFINS, PASTA, HOT DOG AND HAMBURGER BUNS, AND PIZZA DOUGH

These foods contain flour and very little else. A slice of bread has about 15 grams of carb, a cup of cooked spaghetti has 40 grams of carb, and a slice of thin-crust 16-inch pizza has 30 grams of carb.

COOKIES, CAKES, PASTRIES, MUFFINS, AND DONUTS

These foods contain both sugar and flours, and so are sources of sweet and starch. A frosted donut has 20 grams of sugar and 40 grams of carbohydrate.

BASIC CONCEPT #3: TIMING MATTERS: THE MORNING CORTISOL PULSE

For most of our evolutionary history we did not simply roll out of bed and pop a frozen waffle into the toaster. We had to get out and work pretty hard to find something to eat. Nature helps us accomplish all that by designing our hormonal cycles so that we're fully charged with energy in the morning. One of the key hormone cycles for making this happen is the morning cortisol pulse.

Cortisol's job is to free up energy for our brain to figure out how to get food and for our muscles to track our food down. In fact, many people feel no hunger when they wake up in the morning and really don't even want breakfast, but they've heard the myth about needing to "rev up" their metabolism for the day, so they force themselves to eat. Usually they'll eat something "light," which means low in fat and high in sugar or starchy carb.

What the breakfast-is-the-most-important-meal-of-the-day proponents do not realize is that breakfast is actually the worst time of day to eat starchy carb and sugar because doing so will spike your insulin, and cortisol and insulin have opposite effects. Cortisol is all about burning fat and giving you energy. Insulin is all about building fat and making you sleepy.

Eating carbs in the morning will force your body to release MORE insulin to control your blood sugar level than if you ate those carbs later in the day. If you wait to eat your carbs later in the day, you'll typically have considerably less cortisol in your body, and your body can release a good deal less insulin. Since cortisol levels decline later in the day, the later in the day you have your carbs, the better. So instead of a bagel for breakfast, have pizza for dinner. Instead of a banana in the morning, have a little fruit or slightly sweetened dressing with your dinner salad to help those healthy foods taste more delicious.

There's another reason evening is the best time to enjoy your carbs. If you've been active during the day, especially if you have an active job or you work out, your body's sugar storage compartments have been emptied out at least in part thanks to your activity. These storage compartments are located in your muscles and your liver, and they're called *glycogen* granules. Think of them as tiny suitcases for sugar.

In the morning those suitcases are stuffed full because you've been lying down sleeping all night. By evening, however, they've been partly emptied out and so have room to accept whatever sugar comes from your food. This clears your bloodstream of sugar faster so you don't get a blood sugar spike.

When your sugar suitcases are ready to suck sugar from your bloodstream, you release less insulin. So carb consumed at night has less of a fat-building impact, whether consumed in the form of fruit or slow-digesting carb—or even your typical dessert foods, like cookies and ice cream.

So when it comes to carbs, procrastination is a good thing because putting off carbohydrate until later in the day is better than being a carb early bird. Knowing how time of day can turn friendly carbohydrates into the enemy of fatburn is going to help you as you go through each phase of the plan.

WHAT'S A HEALTHY AMOUNT OF SUGAR IN THE BLOOD? LESS THAN A TEASPOON.

If a normal blood sugar level is 100 and a diabetic has a blood sugar level of 300, you might think their blood would be so sugary it would be thick and sweet like syrup. But that's not the case. The body regulates the sugar content of blood so effectively that even poorly controlled diabetics still don't carry that much sugar in their blood. A blood sugar level of 100 in an average height adult translates to 3 to 4 grams of sugar, which is less than a teaspoon. When you lose your ability to send fat to your brain in the form of ketones and it becomes dependent on sugar, the amount of energy it gets is dramatically reduced. And this makes you tired and hungry more often.

As you learned in Chapter 3 (The Diabetes Spectrum), hypoglycemia is the first condition on the diabetes spectrum, when your brain becomes dependent on sugar and forces your liver to raise your blood sugar levels. But that additional sugar stimulates insulin release from the pancreas, initiating the deterioration of the mechanisms that keep your blood sugar in perfect balance.

The way a healthy body keeps our sugar so tightly regulated is efficient and logical. The process starts even before sugar enters our blood, as the body prepares to begin distributing and storing calories the moment we begin to digest any food.

We have taste receptors for sweetness in the gut that are exactly like taste buds on our tongue, except that they are wired to different organs on the other end of the nerves. Taste buds in our brain are hooked up to the appetite regulation center, and help to set our cravings. Taste buds in the gut stimulate hormone release, including the hormone insulin.

INSULIN REDUCES BLOOD SUGAR BY BUILDING FAT

Insulin's job is to get glucose sugar out of your bloodstream and into storage ASAP.

There are only three places in our body that store sugar: muscle, liver, and fat. Muscle and liver store sugar mostly in the form of a kind of starch, called *glycogen*. Both muscle and liver keep glycogen in granules that are like little tiny suitcases of starch. But fat does not have these tiny suitcases and it can't store any glycogen at all. Fat stores sugar in the form of fat.

Insulin stimulates fat cells to take in sugar from your bloodstream. Sugar and fat are completely different molecules, so your body fat can't store sugar. It has to convert it into fat first, using specialized enzymes within the fat cell that reshape sugar's carbon atoms one by one, separating and rearranging them, in order to build them into a fat molecule. The reason this is a useful exercise for the body has to do with the fact that fat is not as sticky as sugar, so your body's cells can store more of it. Fat is also more energy-dense, so you can pack way more calories into a smaller space.

While insulin helps turn sugar into body fat, there's no single hormone that reverses the trick, and that means there's no easy way for your body to undo the process and convert fat back into sugar. This is yet another reason it's so important for you to be able to burn body fat because once you've turned sugar into fat, there's no easy way of turning it back.

Unfortunately for those of us who love our sweets and starches, as long as there's more than just a trace of insulin in the bloodstream, we cannot easily burn body fat. Why not? Because insulin shuts down the enzymes that release body fat into the bloodstream. If your insulin level is much above baseline, then your body fat is going to stay trapped in your adipose tissue, where it's unable to provide your cells with energy. If losing weight has become harder than it used to be, and a minor lapse in your discipline opens the gates and weight comes flooding back into your body, that is a sign that your insulin level might be high all the time, keeping your fat locked in storage and making it very hard for you to lose any excess weight. This condition is called insulin resistance.

INSULIN RESISTANCE: TOO MUCH INSULIN ALL THE TIME

As you learned in Chapter 3 (The Diabetes Spectrum), insulin resistance typically develops around the time a person first starts to notice they gain weight easier than they used to, sometimes with a first pregnancy or the birth of a child.

Once you've become insulin-resistant, eating anything sweet or starchy makes your insulin go much higher than normal and keeps your insulin high for a longer-than-normal amount of time. This not only keeps your body fat locked in storage; it also blocks your liver's ability to make ketones for your brain. Without the ability to make ketones from your body fat, your brain is overly dependent on sugar, and many folks with insulin resistance find they need to snack to keep their energy up. Another common sign you might have insulin resistance is that when you eat a very sweet or starchy meal, like pancakes for breakfast or a soda, a sandwich, and chips for lunch, you get tired a couple hours later.

Folks with even mild insulin resistance often find it very hard to lose weight while continuing to eat starchy carbs and sweets because each infusion of carbohydrate from the breakfast oatmeal or the lunchtime power bar or the afternoon banana or dinnertime pasta and desserts bumps up their insulin again. When you're insulin-resistant, your body needs to release more insulin to get the same job done, so your insulin levels go higher after you eat a given amount of carbohydrate than if you were not insulin-resistant. The higher your insulin level climbs, the longer it takes to fall. It can take so long to fall that even after your blood sugar level is back to your baseline level, your fat remains locked in storage, and when your cells cry out for energy there's simply none to be found. This is why people with insulin resistance often notice feeling tired an hour or two after eating a high-carb meal.

When you google "what causes insulin resistance," you'll find a variety of answers, but what they all more or less agree on is that inflammation has something to do with it. The advice you'll get from these well-meaning bloggers is all over the map. You'll read folks telling you that to reduce inflammation in your body you'll need to eat only organic foods, avoid dairy, gluten, lectins, high-fructose corn syrup, GMOs, glyphosate herbicide, and on and on. But none of that is accurate.

The information from doctors is not much clearer. Different experts have come up with a variety of explanations for the cause of insulin resistance. Some blame too much saturated fat. Others say it's not fat but sugar that causes insulin resistance. Another group says it's lack of exercise. And still others say insulin resistance is simply how your body tries to adapt to weight gain. The theory here is that depending on your genetics, the amount of body fat you build can exceed a threshold where it can no longer accommodate storing anything more. This is the "personal fat threshold" theory of insulin resistance.

But the reality is that it's not milk or gluten or your genetics that cause insulin resistance. The dramatic shift in the chemical nature of your body fat is the most likely cause.

Insulin resistance is a result of a metabolic one-two punch. As I've argued, the first punch comes from vegetable oil, which damages your mitochondria so your brain grows dependent on sugar. And the second punch comes from your brain forcing your liver to pump out more sugar than your blood is designed to safely carry. This mismatch between energy supply and ancient blood-sugar-regulating physiologic rules pits your liver and pancreas against each other in a never-ending battle.

Aside from making us build fat, insulin also helps our body know there's nutrition around. Whenever a person eats anything, a little bit of insulin gets released. When we eat something high in sugar or starch, we release a lot more. After a healthy person eats a candy bar or a cookie, insulin might spike quickly from a level of, say, 1.5 or 2 mIU/L to maybe 30 or 50 mIU/L, then within minutes come back down. With insulin resistance, the person's pre-snack insulin level is usually well above 10 mIU/L, and after a candy bar or a cookie it can soar to 100 or 200 mIU/L or even higher. Insulin spikes like these may accelerate insulin resistance, so eliminating your intake of starch and sugar is an essential part of treating every disease on the diabetes spectrum.

HOW LOW SHOULD YOU GO?

Most low-carb doctors will tell you that you don't need any carb at all because your body can make its own sugar out of protein. That's true: your liver can make sugar from protein. But forcing your liver to make sugar from protein is not a good idea. I don't agree that we should cut our carbs out altogether until you know your body can burn at least a little bit of fat for you.

The reason I disagree with cutting out all carbs right off the bat, as low-carb and keto diet books typically recommend, has to do with the reality that some folks are not able to do it safely. The problem with jumping headfirst into a low-carb diet before you're ready is that you are at high risk of suffering from hypoglycemia symptoms. Remember the eleven symptoms? Hypoglycemia symptoms occur so often when starting a low-carb diet they've come to be called the "low-carb flu" (similarly, the "keto flu" is associated with keto diets).

These symptoms sometimes disappear after pushing through for a few days, but I'm not OK with that strategy. Firstly, as we learned in Chapter 1, hypoglycemia symptoms can occasionally cause ministrokes, leaving permanent scars in the brain. Secondly, the symptoms may improve simply because the liver is converting protein to sugar faster than ever—thus worsening your metabolic problems. Furthermore, some people's negative experience convinces them that their body is wired to need more carbs than other people's, and that's simply not true. A healthy metabolism can handle a huge range of carb intakes, all the way down to zero.

Just as hypoglycemia symptoms should be recognized as a metabolic problem and properly treated, so should the low-carb flu. The trouble is, folks with frequent hypoglycemia are in a bind because they do need to cut carbs to reduce insulin spikes and insulin resistance, but when they go ahead and cut their carbs, instead of feeling the energy they'd hoped for, they feel really bad.

Wouldn't it be great if there was a way you could take in moderate amounts of carbs so that you could avoid these symptoms while at the same time avoiding insulin spikes and start to heal your hormone systems?

Good news. There is!

SCIENCE BOX: WHAT'S A HEALTHY INSULIN LEVEL?

The standard lab will tell you that a fasting insulin level under 25 mIU/L is normal. This is way too high; so many people are insulin-resistant that it's skewed the statistics so that average levels are higher than what's healthy.

It doesn't take much insulin to stop your body's fat cells from releasing fat. At a blood insulin level of roughly 1 mIU/L, your fat cells can release fat at 80 to 90 percent of your maximal (maximal is actually a moving target because a highly trained athlete will release more than a person who never exercises, and things like cortisol and adrenaline boost fat release). At a blood insulin level of just 10, that number plummets, dipping to around 5 percent of maximal. Most normal-weight, healthy Americans who exercise on a regular basis have insulin levels around 1.5 or 2 first thing in the morning. The typical overweight patient of mine has a level somewhere around 7 to 15, meaning they wake up after burning mostly sugar all night and are already running low on cellular fuel so that if they don't have time for breakfast, they'll rarely be able to make it all the way to lunch without feeling weak.

SCIENCE SOAPBOX: HELP RAISE AWARENESS OF INSULIN RESISTANCE

Given the far-reaching consequences of insulin resistance, many low-carb doctors, including myself, find it absurd that standard medical practice totally overlooks the condition. We should be considering hormonal problems the minute someone comes in experiencing hypoglycemia. Instead, standard practice is for doctors to ignore insulin resistance and wait until problems progress all the way to prediabetes and sometimes even to diabetes before ever giving people a diagnosis or a hint that something is wrong. Don't expect this to change any time soon because the American Medical Association has yet to provide a unique diagnosis code for insulin resistance so doctors can at least recognize it as a disease. Without a diagnostic code, those few doctors who do understand insulin resistance can't make a proper recording of this serious problem in your medical chart.

What should you do to raise awareness of this problem? I wish I had an easy answer for this one. Unfortunately, unless you're a media spokesperson specializing in health or in a leadership position in the healthcare industry, there's not much you can do at this time. Just focus on healing yourself.

BLACK BOX WARNING: DON'T CUT CARBS WITHOUT LEARNING HOW TO ADJUST YOUR MEDICATIONS

If you are a diabetic and take insulin or other drugs that lower your blood sugar, then going low-carb without knowing how to adjust your medications can put you at serious risk. When you cut your carbs, you reduce your need for insulin significantly. If you continue to use the same dose, you can drop your blood sugar so low that you get a serious hypoglycemia reaction, and some people can even pass out. A famous case of attempted murder in the 1980s involved a husband intentionally overdosing his wife with insulin—that's how serious hypoglycemia can be. You definitely want to work with a doctor to adjust your medications downward. Even if your doctor is not a fan of low-carb diets and won't help you with this process, you can search online for find a low-carb practitioner in your area or available virtually who will help walk you through this process.

SCIENCE SOAPBOX: TREATING TYPE 2 DIABETICS WITH INSULIN IS UNETHICAL

If you or anyone you know is using insulin to treat their type 2 diabetes, you might be surprised to learn that insulin itself can make you more insulin-resistant and that when you use insulin to lower your blood sugar, you're making your metabolic problems worse. Even though all doctors know that type 2 diabetics are insulin-resistant and that injecting more insulin into their bodies will accelerate their weight gain, it's still currently standard of care to prescribe insulin for type 2 diabetes. Once a practice has become standard of care, it takes decades or longer to change.

DR. CATE'S SLOW CARB SOLUTION TO THE LOW-CARB FLU

Most low-carbohydrate and keto dieters restrict all carbohydrates, without making a distinction between carbs that are refined and those that are unrefined. The distinction matters because nature often encapsulates carbs with a kind of time-release structure, thus blunting the spikes that block fatburning. Refining removes these structures, exposing you to blood sugar spikes that you don't experience when the natural time-release structures remain intact.

Foods like beans, nuts, and intact whole grains—not whole grain flours—won't spike your sugar or your insulin thanks to the fact that they're encapsulated in indigestible cellulose, accompanied by fat or protein or both. The cellulose, fat, and protein all serve to slow down the process of digestion, so that instead of rushing into your bloodstream, causing a big spike, the sugar dribbles into your bloodstream slowly. That way, you can get enough sugar to avoid the low-carb flu but not so much that it causes problems.

I call these time-release foods the "slow carbs."

You'll be using slow carbs during Phase I of the plan. Slow carbs smooth your transition from a higher-carb to a lower-carb diet, allowing chronically high insulin levels to settle down. Slow carbs represent a key piece

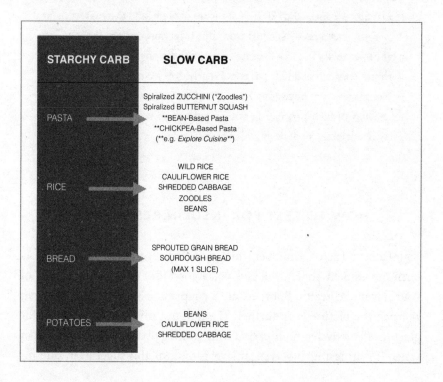

STARCHY CARB	SLOW CARB
PASTA	Spiralized ZUCCHINI ("Zoodles") Spiralized BUTTERNUT SQUASH **BEAN-Based Pasta **CHICKPEA-Based Pasta (**e.g. *Explore Cuisine***)
RICE	WILD RICE CAULIFLOWER RICE SHREDDED CABBAGE ZOODLES BEANS
BREAD	SPROUTED GRAIN BREAD SOURDOUGH BREAD (MAX 1 SLICE)
POTATOES	BEANS CAULIFLOWER RICE SHREDDED CABBAGE

of the necessary metabolic-rehabilitation process, and one that most diets overlook.

WHAT'S A MACRO?

"Macro" is Greek for "big," and in the world of nutrition "macro" is short for "macronutrient." Macronutrients are the three categories of "big" nutrients: proteins, carbohydrates, and fats. Many diets are defined by their macros: high-carb, low-fat, high-protein. The specific proportion of calories of each macro serves as a quick way to compare and contrast different diets. Most popular diets focus more on one macronutrient and provide less detail about the others. The popular low-carb diets usually contain less than 20 percent of calories from carbohydrates, with keto going as low as 10 percent. Low-fat diets often contain as little as 10 percent of calories from fat. Dietitians wedded to the standard orthodoxy recommend a so-called "balanced" diet, and their somewhat off-center definition of "balance" means a majority of calories from carbohydrates (45 to 65 percent), 15 to 20 percent from protein, and the rest from fat.

As you can already see just from this brief description, there's quite a bit of variability in carbohydrate recommendations. The macronutrient with the least variability is protein. Nearly every diet suggests a protein intake somewhere between 15 and 20 percent of daily calories, with the exception of high-protein diets that push it up to 35 percent—often using proprietary protein-powder blends.

HOW TO TEST FOR INSULIN RESISTANCE

Your Fatburn Factor, a number which we will determine in Chapter 9 (Fatburn Assessment Tools), will give you a good idea of the current state of your metabolic health. But there are a couple of laboratory tests that can sharpen the picture even further. The first test involves a blood test for glucose after a twelve-hour period with nothing to eat or drink other than water. If your fasting blood sugar level is over 90, this suggests insulin resistance, but it is not the most sensitive test and many people with insulin levels in the 80s already have insulin resistance.

For a more definitive answer, you can use a few other tools based on a few other simple blood tests.

One is called the HOMA-IR, and you need a fasting glucose and a fasting insulin level to calculate it. You calculate your HOMA-IR by plugging the glucose and insulin levels into a simple formula: take the glucose value, multiply it by the insulin value, and divide that by 405. The result is called your *homeostatic model assessment of insulin resistance*, or HOMA-IR score. You can also find HOMA-IR calculators online to do the math for you: all you do is plug in the glucose and insulin numbers. A result of less than 1.0 means you are insulin-sensitive, which is optimal. Above 1.9 indicates early insulin resistance. Above 2.9 indicates significant insulin resistance.

Another test of insulin resistance is the triglyceride-to-HDL ratio. A standard fasting cholesterol panel includes these numbers. To calculate, simply divide the triglyceride number on your report by the HDL number. If the result is under 2, you're in pretty good shape. If it's under 1, you're in very good shape. If it's over 2.5, that's a strong indication of insulin resistance. Between 2 and 2.5 is probable insulin resistance.

Many low-carb doctors, including myself, find it useful to conduct a more complicated test to better gauge the degree of insulin resistance. The protocol involves drinking a known quantity of sugar and then retesting your glucose and insulin anywhere from one to five hours after finishing the drink. Some doctors like to test at hourly intervals, but I find you can get a lot of information just by testing at the two-hour time point. A resulting insulin level above 60 suggests problems. A level of 150 or higher is clearly problematic. Numbers in the 200s and 300s are not unheard of and suggest that you may be resistant to hormones other than insulin.

Insulin is the canary in the coal mine of hormone resistance. In other words, if you're resistant to insulin, that is a good indicator that you may be losing sensitivity to other hormones as well. That's why I would suggest that anyone who has thyroid disease, low testosterone, leptin resistance, infertility, or irregular periods consider getting some assessment of their insulin sensitivity.

If you suffer from hormone-resistance problems, whether those hormone levels are normal or not, fixing your fatburn will very likely improve your hormone function and your symptoms. In fact, fixing your fatburn sometimes works even better than taking hormone replacements. In my experience, most men with low T who get shots experience initial symptom improvement, but after three months the effect wears off. However, those who fix their fatburn often normalize their testosterone levels without shots and experience lasting benefits in testosterone function.

The far-reaching benefits of improving insulin sensitivity are becoming better recognized by some of the more forward-thinking gynecologists, and it's now common practice to treat infertility and PCOS with a low-carb diet before offering hormonal therapies.

Given that your ability to respond to insulin is a critical piece of the health-recovery puzzle, and such a good indicator of your long-term health future, I feel that a fasting insulin level should be built into the labs done with an annual physical along with the cholesterol panel. Everyone should know their HOMA-IR and triglyceride-to-HDL ratio just as they know their weight and height.

SCIENCE BOX: LOW-CARB OR KETO CAN RAISE CHOLESTEROL. SO WHAT?

What I love most about the low-carb and keto diets is that they encourage people to eat traditional fats like butter, coconut, bacon, and cheese. When you eat a lot of these traditional, healthy fats, insulin tells the liver to pack that fat into giant particles called *very low-density lipoprotein*, or VLDL. VLDL carries lots of cholesterol, and high VLDL will raise your total cholesterol, which is true whether you have insulin resistance or not. This is why a keto diet can also raise your doctor's eyebrows, because most doctors are still programmed to believe that cholesterol causes heart attacks.

Those of us who study the issue more closely, however, do not fear high cholesterol.

When you cut carbs and eat more healthy fats, you raise your HDL cholesterol—and that's a good thing. All doctors, even the most drug-loving, cholesterol-fearing cardiologists, agree that high HDL is better than low HDL. Low HDL is actually one of the strongest predictors of heart attack. When your HDL goes up, so do your total cholesterol levels.

What's more, when you start burning your body fat, your LDL often goes up. The companies who sell LDL-lowering pharmaceuticals have spent billions of dollars brainwashing doctors into being terrified of high LDL. But the fact is, we shouldn't be. High LDL is correlated with higher IQ, greater longevity, improved memory, and less chance of dying from cancer or infection. For more on the topic of cholesterol and heart disease, see the resources section.

INSULIN RESISTANCE ROBS YOUR BODY OF KETONES

In order for your liver to make ketones, your insulin must be low. Folks with insulin resistance will have high insulin levels most of the day, leaving the liver little to no opportunity to make ketones.

Now that you know how much your brain loves ketones, you can guess that the high insulin levels associated with insulin resistance present a particular problem for your brain. While other tissues can more easily switch to burning dietary fat—the fat from your last meal—the brain, surrounded by the blood-brain barrier that blocks access to most dietary fats, must rely on sugar when there are no ketones around.

Remember, your brain uses up 20 percent of your total resting energy. This means that if you have insulin resistance, you actually have a higher dietary requirement for sugar than if you have a healthy metabolism.

You might be wondering, if the brain loves ketones so much, why doesn't the liver just make ketones all the time? The reality is that, given a healthy metabolism and a diet low in refined carbs and sugars, your liver makes a lot of ketones a lot of the time. This feeds into a virtuous cycle of rapidly improved health and opportunity for weight loss, because the more ketones your liver makes, the less hunger you experience and the less often you need to eat. Eating less often allows your liver to pump out ketones for a larger proportion of the time, giving you more energy to be more active, burn more fat, and accelerate your weight loss.

So now you know that if you cut clean-burning, natural fat, you are driven to seek sugar and starchy carbohydrates, which can make you hungry and tired. Not only are we driven to rely on sugar due to vegetable-oil-induced mitochondrial damage, we're driven to consume foods that disrupt our hormonal systems and make us overeat.

Next, we'll take a look at the component of your metabolism that's truly the star of this book, your body fat, and discover what happens to you when your body fat contains too much unstable vegetable oil.

7

Fatburn System 3

Your Body Fat

IN THIS CHAPTER YOU'LL LEARN

- Toxic amounts of polyunsaturated fat make your body fat dysfunctional.
- Dysfunctional body fat causes fat buildup in your arteries and organs.
- Blood tests and certain symptoms help you recognize body fat dysfunction.

Most of us think of body fat as a kind of useless collection of gooey material that we carry around all day, whose main function seems to be to make our clothes bulge out in a variety of unattractive ways. A more complete understanding of body fat comes only when you think of it as a living dynamic tissue, like an organ. Medically speaking, it actually is an organ, meeting every definition of the term: it's a group of tissues in a living organism that has been adapted to perform a specific function. Just like other organs, body fat can be healthy, or it can get sick and fail to serve its functions.

One of the jobs body fat is designed to do is store fat. Another is to release fat. In this chapter, we'll be looking at how a diet of pro-inflammatory oils can make both of these two equally important functions of your body fat go haywire.

To lay the groundwork for that discussion, we'll go through the process of building fat when your metabolism is perfectly healthy. This is important so you can understand that eating too much of any kind of food—even healthy foods—forces you to build fat. In other words, yes, calories do count. Once we understand how healthy body fat is supposed to behave, we will be better positioned to understand the health problems that can crop up when your body fat is not working correctly.

THE CALORIE CLOSET

You may look at your body fat in the mirror and think it's just sitting there doing nothing, but looks can be deceiving. Right now, as you're reading this, your body fat is busy doing one of two things: either building fat out of food you recently ingested or releasing fat into your bloodstream so that your cells have a chance to burn it. When you gain weight, it's because your body fat is building more than you burn. When you lose weight, it's because your body fat is releasing more than it builds.

Your body fat is called *adipose* to distinguish it from dietary fat. (I could have called this book *The Adiposeburn Fix*, for example, to be more technically correct.) Most of your adipose tissue is located under your skin, where it's easy to see how much you've accumulated. We also have small amounts of adipose fat around our internal organs for cushioning. A man or woman of healthy weight carries about 100,000 calories in storage in their adipose, enough to run the four hundred miles from LA to San Francisco in forty-eight hours without refueling, or go for weeks without eating should the need ever arise.

Think of all this body fat as a kind of closet where you store energy from your last meal. We previously saw that any sugar, fat, or protein that exceeds your body's need will be converted, with insulin's help, into space-saving molecules of fat. Here, I want to emphasize a common point of confusion about protein. You may have heard that protein triggers muscle growth, and that may have given you the impression that calories in protein-rich foods or protein powders won't make you build fat. But the fact is, extra protein beyond what your body requires at any given time will be converted into fat. For most nonathletes, protein shakes and bars and foods that jack your daily protein intake beyond 70 to 100 grams or so are not going to wind up in your muscle. Instead, the additional protein will end up piling on to your body fat.

In order for you to be able to burn body fat off, the first step is to release fat from the closet. We already saw that low insulin levels enable your body fat to release stored fat in the form of *free fatty acids*. With insulin at low levels, this allows the doors to the calorie closet to swing open, releasing free fatty acids into the bloodstream. Insulin being low is actually a key to all the metabolic activities involved in burning body fat. In other words, you need to get your insulin levels down before you can easily burn body fat.

Once those free fatty acids have entered the bloodstream, they can gain access to every part of your body that might be needing energy. If there is no need for energy, the body removes free fatty acids from the bloodstream in a timely manner. If a free fatty acid is not scooped up by a hungry cell in need of energy in about two minutes, it will be scooped up by the liver, which plays a key role in regulating the fuels available in your bloodstream.

What the liver does with those fatty acids depends on your insulin levels. While insulin stays low and the body remains in fatburning mode, the liver will chop up the fatty acid to make ketones. Remember, ketones are a preferred fuel for almost every organ in your body. So even when your metabolism is healthy, you won't make ketones unless your insulin levels are low, and without ketones you're going to feel hungry more often. Low insulin is therefore essential to controlling hunger.

Whenever insulin levels rise for any reason, the liver shifts gears, converting from fatburning to fat building. When the liver is in fat-building mode, the free fatty acids arriving at the liver will be packed it into a special fat-transport vehicle called a *lipoprotein*. The lipoprotein travels through the bloodstream, delivering fat to all your tissues. While insulin is high, the body tends to use any fat it gets for the purposes of building new cells rather than burning for energy. And if a lipoprotein is not snapped up by any tissue, then after a short while—usually a matter of hours—it will end up back in your body fat.

In other words, insulin controls whether fat released from the calorie closet will be burned for energy or stored in the calorie closet again. And this is why for your metabolism to remain efficient and flexible, for your calorie closet to function flawlessly—opening and closing its doors in response to hormonal instructions to either accept fat from the bloodstream for storage or to release fat back into the bloodstream to be used for fuel—you must have normal insulin levels and normal insulin sensitivity.

There are actually a host of hormones other than insulin that play a role in controlling whether the calorie closet is accepting calories and building fat or releasing calories to be burned as fuel. Hormones like glucagon, adrenaline, human growth hormone, thyroid hormone, estrogen, testosterone, and many more. The reason we have so many hormones weighing in on whether your calorie closet should be storing or releasing its fuel is to ensure that all the different body tissues that might need fat for fuel have access to their share. It's a massive coordination effort, and hormone signaling is one of the key methods of coordinating the body's ever-changing energy needs.

For your metabolism to function properly, it needs to respond to all these various hormone signals quickly and accurately. In the last chapter, we saw how inflammation gets in the way of signal transmission. And where is inflammation coming from? By now, you know the answer: vegetable oil, loaded with inflammation-promoting and dangerously unstable fats. Next, we're going to take a look at the impact of inflammation on your body fat and discover what happens when the largest organ in your body fails to do its job.

THE DYSFUNCTIONAL CALORIE CLOSET

In the past two chapters, we've learned that inflammation driven by unstable fats in vegetable oil causes dysfunction in each of the two fatburn systems we've already discussed. Now we're ready to explore the idea that this inflammation—and not saturated fat, cholesterol, or even carbohydrates in moderation—makes wayward body fat accumulate around your waist, causing belly fat, and in your arteries, causing heart attacks and strokes.

Belly Fat

Obesity researchers have given us a new understanding of obesity, that there are actually two kinds. There is a relatively healthy kind, what doctors call *metabolically healthy obesity*. And there is the unhealthy kind, associated with inflammation.

As the largest organ in your body, your body fat has a big responsibility. It must be able to coordinate energy storage and release in service of all the other organs of the body, no matter what you eat, how active you are, the time of day, how much sleep you get, and so on. Your body fat communicates with all other body tissues by way of hormones and cytokines, those it makes and those it releases.

You may be one of those lucky people with a big happy family that stays in touch all the time, not just on holidays but calling daily, sharing photos on Facebook, Skyping on weekends or evenings instead of watching TV, or, if you're really old-school, sending postcards when you go on vacation. All your organs are supposed to be just like that big happy family, communicating through various hormones, the biological equivalent of social media and iPhones. Just as these tools help your family plan dinners and get-togethers, hormones help coordinate your body's complex functions.

To keep the other parts of your body up to date on what's going on with your adipose, your body fat produces its own set of hormones, in the neighborhood of fifty different kinds. Your body fat must also respond to external hormones produced by every other organ. When your body fat gets sick and inflamed from a lifetime of toxic vegetable oil consumption, hormone responsiveness declines, and the coordination process can't function properly.

Obesity researchers now recognize there are two entirely different kinds of obesity with entirely different health consequences. The two different types of obesity are distinguished by whether the coordination process functions efficiently and thus enables you to more safely deal with the problem of excess body fat. Those people with healthy body fat are called metabolically healthy obese, and those with unhealthy body fat are called metabolically unhealthy obese.

The differences are easy to spot—you can tell simply by looking at where a person's body builds the extra fat.

If you are in the metabolically healthy category, your body is better able to accommodate more fat. This means you are a person who puts their fat in "all the right places," maintaining an hourglass silhouette. Your need to store additional fat can be fulfilled by the adipose tissue located under your skin, called *subcutaneous* body fat ("subcutaneous" means "under skin"), which is supposed to be the primary place our excess calories are stored. Healthy adipose tissue easily accommodates additional shipments of fat by reproducing new baby fat cells, called preadipocytes. Preadipocytes, in turn, respond to the hormones adiponectin and insulin, as well as other hormones, by maturing into fully functioning members of the adipocyte community.

The happy side of being able to create new fat cells on demand this way is that it relieves the existing fat cells of having to take on more fat than they would like to, which leads to a healthier form of body fat that is not itself inflamed and does not contribute to inflammatory problems elsewhere in the body. Folks with this form of obesity are generally free from common problems typically associated with obesity like diabetes, hypertension, kidney disease, gout, and fatty liver. The downside of having such accommodating, responsive fat cells is that it means you put on weight very easily.

The other option when faced with the need to store fat is to simply shove more into the existing collection of cells, making each individual cell abnormally fat. This adaptation is associated with insulin resistance, abnormal adiponectin levels, and a tendency to develop central or "truncal" obesity. When I see someone with a beer gut, skinny legs, or fat under their chin around their neck, I know that their metabolism isn't healthy and therefore neither is their fat. This pattern of weight distribution is the external sign of an internal disruption in fat distribution that is further revealed by the fact that people with this body type tend to have lab abnormalities indicating risk of heart attack and stroke, including high triglycerides, low HDL, and elevated liver enzymes.

Additionally, when you've overburdened your fat cells with too great a load of storage fat, your body fat can become inflamed to the point it actually hurts. I've seen this in a few patients with fibromyalgia who developed hard and tender nodules in their fat, and I can tell you that the pain people with this condition suffer from can be agonizing.

Chronically overstuffed fat cells may also release distress signals, called *adipokines*, into the bloodstream. Adipokines can be measured with a simple blood test, and if your adipokines are high, some research suggests you may be at higher risk of blood clots as well as certain cancers.

Whether you remain metabolically healthy or develop metabolically unhealthy body fat may be determined by your genes. Those people with less advantageous genetics gain little body fat, but right off the bat develop belly fat and a double chin. Those with more advantageous genetics can gain much more weight before things start to look out of proportion. Regardless of your genetics and your body type, your body fat will function better as the proportion of toxic vegetable oils in your diet declines.

So we've seen that fat cells full of vegetable oil become inflamed and stop cooperating with the rest of the family. But you really do need to forgive these misbehaving fat cells because it's absolutely not their fault that they've been behaving so passive-aggressively. While other cells can say no to shipments of pro-inflammatory fat and request extra sugar for fuel instead, the fat cells are dealing with more inflammation all the time for the benefit of the rest of the body. In fact, pro-inflammatory fat is generating so much inflammation that it attracts about thirty times more white blood cells than normal. So it's almost like the fat cells are suffering from a chronic infection.

When rejected by overstuffed fat cells, the orphaned triglyceride can also infiltrate otherwise lean tissues like liver and bone; this is called ectopic fat. This next section will touch on the real cause of most arterial disease, which originates not in foods like butter and eggs, as we so often hear (and as I was taught in medical school), but in orphaned triglyceride that's been rejected by every other tissue and has no permanent place to call home.

YOUR BODY FAT REMEMBERS

Your body fat is like Vegas: what happens in your body fat stays in your body fat—at least for quite a long time.

As we've discussed, your fat closet reflects the fatty acid content of the foods you've eaten. If you've spent a lot of time eating foods with vegetable oil as a major ingredient—mayonnaise, chips, fried foods, store-bought salad dressings—then the fat you've stored away in your fat closet reflects the fatty acid content of vegetable oils. In that sense, your body fat keeps a record of what you've eaten in the past. On the TV series *Game of Thrones*, "The North remembers" is an oft-repeated phrase among the Northerners. It means that the Northerners don't easily forget past events, especially betrayals. Your body fat is the same way. After you stop eating vegetable oil, it can take months before those remnants of long-ago meals have been eliminated from your body.

Fat Spills in Your Arteries

The narrative of insulin resistance naturally dovetails into the story of arterial disease, and leads to one of its life-threatening complications: the fatty plaques that build up in blood vessels to cause heart attacks and strokes. This is because another consequence of overburdening fat cells with more than they can handle is that, at some point, they simply can't take on any more. In other words, even though the hormone insulin is telling them to hurry up and clear triglyceride from the bloodstream, they have no choice but to disobey insulin's order, leaving abnormally high levels of circulating triglyceride in your bloodstream.

The most worrisome complication of insulin resistance is that the excess triglyceride in your circulatory system can start to deposit along the walls of your arteries, leading to arteriosclerosis—the plaques that cause heart attacks and strokes.

When the concentration of unstable fatty acids stored in your individual fat cells reaches a critical threshold, your body fat can no longer readily perform one of its chief functions: building new stores of body fat. When triglyceride and sugar can't gain access to your body fat, they stay in the bloodstream, promoting the development of plaque in your arteries. This in a nutshell is the cause of heart attacks and strokes.

Let's take a slightly more detailed look at how insulin-resistant fat cells, unable to welcome new deliveries with open arms, lead to the development of arterial plaque to see how it compares to the standard explanation you'll hear in a doctor's office—and why that currently accepted explanation actually makes no physiologic sense.

LIPOPROTEINS: FEDEX FOR FAT

Lipoproteins are spherical structures composed of fat and protein (lipo + protein) that transport fat through your arteries. If your doctor tells you your "bad" cholesterol is too high, he's talking about a fat-delivery vehicle known as low-density lipoprotein, or LDL cholesterol. LDL cholesterol is not "bad," in spite of what most people say.

Why would your doctor tell you something that's not true? Because the science we ourselves learn is corrupted by bias. Here I need to digress for a moment to reframe what you've probably heard about cholesterol all your life.

No area of medicine has been more corrupted by bias than the field of preventive cardiology. Doctors don't get the full story on what really causes heart disease, and most of what you'll be told about cholesterol in any doctor's office is incorrect, even at places like the Cleveland Clinic, Stanford, Yale, and Harvard. So what I'm going to tell you will probably be new, but hopefully it will make more intuitive sense than the claim that cholesterol clogs arteries. By "intuitive sense," I mean that if you know just a little bit of the basics, then common sense should tell you whether or not the claim that cholesterol clogs arteries can possibly be true.

Most of the cholesterol in our bodies is not from our food. It's made by our cells. Our bodies make cholesterol for a reason: every cell in your body requires cholesterol for its membranes, and without cholesterol in our cell membranes, we'd die. Cholesterol is also the building block of a number of important hormones, including testosterone, estrogen, and cortisol. Those facts alone should raise your eyebrows.

Most doctors think eating cholesterol makes our cholesterol go up. That's not true. You might be surprised to learn that one of the most powerful factors causing elevated cholesterol is burning body fat, as that makes your LDL cholesterol go up. Another factor elevating your cholesterol is eating whole foods that are naturally high in fat, especially saturated and monounsaturated fats, which makes your HDL cholesterol go up.

Doctors are taught that LDL gets stuck in your arteries to ultimately cause heart disease, so they call it "bad" cholesterol. And doctors are taught that HDL is like a cholesterol vacuum cleaner, sucking out the cholesterol from your arteries and preventing heart disease, so they call it "good" cholesterol. But these ideas are not representative of accepted lipoprotein physiology. HDL and LDL are simply structures designed to help carry cholesterol and fat in our arteries. The reality is we know that all lipoproteins work in service of the goal of distributing fat and cholesterol throughout the body. You can think of lipoproteins as the body's miniature FedEx delivery vehicles for fat and cholesterol. The difference between all lipoproteins is mostly that they're different sizes, have slightly different compositions and slightly different destinations to which they travel—very much like FedEx has a variety of vehicles: planes, big trucks, and small trucks to cover all of its service areas.

When you carefully examine any one of the mountain of publications that cite cholesterol as the cause of heart disease, you quickly discover the entire argument—which is to say all of preventive cardiology—rests on nothing but a house of cards. Yank away the studies at the bottom—called the Framingham studies—and the whole pile comes crashing down.

More and more doctors, including me, are reviewing the evidence for ourselves and looking at the data directly, not just the summary of the article that's written with drug-company spin. We're finding over and over that the evidence clearly shows that higher LDL is a good thing, associated with less likelihood of dementia, cancer, or infectious disease, and with a prolonged lifespan.

My own LDL cholesterol is 203, way over the so-called upper limit of "normal," which is between 130 and 160, depending on which lab is testing your blood and what year you got it tested. Am I concerned about a heart attack with this high LDL? Not at all. My LDL has gone up since before I changed my diet when I was in my early thirties. Back then, my LDL was much lower because I was not burning my body fat effectively. My metabolism was so unhealthy that I was actually prediabetic with a fasting blood sugar of 113. My vegetable oil consumption was so high that my HDL was 23—extremely low and unhealthy. Now my HDL is 86 and my fasting blood sugar is 85. All these numbers are excellent indicators of insulin sensitivity, healthy lipoproteins, metabolic flexibility, and—most importantly—that my cells are fueling with body fat.

As your fatburn improves, you can use your LDL going up as a good indication that your body is burning more fat.

I hope this brief introduction to the uniquely corrupt science of preventive cardiology gives you a useful perspective and makes you curious enough about the actual cause of heart disease to do a little more digging. For anyone interested in reading more on this topic, see the resources list in the appendix.

Now you understand that toxic vegetable oils in your diet concentrate in your body fat to cause insulin resistance, keeping your body fat stuck on your body and trapping you in a cycle of fatigue, weight gain, and declining health. Vegetable oil in your body fat also suppresses your LDL and HDL, which often rise as your body gets healthier. What you're going to learn next is that the most powerful trap of all, one that puts the biggest barrier in the way of long-term success, is the one in your head.

SCIENCE BOX: WHY MEN START TO DIE FROM HEART ATTACKS TEN YEARS BEFORE WOMEN

As we've seen throughout this chapter, oxygen destabilizes the fatty acids in vegetable oil. Well, the bloodstream has a lot of oxygen, and as the vegetable oil travels in your arterial FedEx trucks, there is a high risk of reacting with oxygen to generate powerfully inflammatory free radical reactions. If lipoproteins are FedEx delivery vehicles delivering fat, the oxygen molecules in your blood are flying bullets that can shoot the tires on the delivery truck, causing accidents that spill triglyceride into the bloodstream. Because men have more oxygen in their blood than women, as well as more iron, which accelerates the reaction, the deposition of fat along the arterial wall happens more quickly, putting men at risk for heart attack and stroke a full ten years earlier than their female counterparts.

8

Fatburn System 4

The Appetite Control Center

IN THIS CHAPTER YOU'LL LEARN

- Your brain's appetite control center matches your calorie intake to your calorie need automatically.
- An inflamed appetite control center cannot do this, making sustained weight loss nearly impossible.
- Rebuilding your brain with healthy fats transforms overactive hunger into cravings for nutrition.

A HEALTHY HUNGER

Hunger is a basic human experience. Yet we are so afraid of it.

You might have heard that you shouldn't allow yourself to feel hunger, as if hunger itself were inherently harmful. You might have heard that being hungry slows your metabolism, and that's why you need to eat first thing in the morning and snack at regular intervals throughout the day. You might have heard that being hungry for too long can put you into a kind of "hibernation" mode or "starvation state" that will make you tired and ultimately make you gain weight. But these assertions are unfounded myths.

The fact is, people who are metabolically healthy do not get hungry unless they've been extremely active, skipped a couple of meals, or have been undereating for a few days in a row. When they do get hungry, the next meal they eat will taste really, really good. As Miguel de Cervantes observed long ago, "Hunger is the best sauce in the world."

Hunger is also a great teacher. In a metabolically healthy person, hunger goes beyond the body's need for energy and awakens the body to its nutritional needs. A healthy hunger is designed to direct us to nutritious foods with savory, salty, and sour flavors. These flavors come from proteins, minerals, and acids that enable us to build lean tissue and help digest our food, and the flavor of all these nutrients is enhanced in the presence of natural fats.

I believe the reason that we fear hunger the way we do is that our experience of hunger is no longer normal. These days so many people are metabolically unhealthy that, as we saw earlier, normal hunger has been replaced by a dangerous kind of hunger. This dangerous hunger can occur just a few hours after eating. And unlike healthy hunger, abnormal hunger is not about getting nutrients. It's about getting sugar into your brain. This abnormal hunger drives unhealthy habits, making you crave sugar in ways that are incompatible with sustained weight loss.

When your metabolism is healthy, your experience of hunger will be very different from what it is right now. Instead of making you tired, it will energize you. Instead of driving you towards junk food, you'll pass over the junk food in search of actual nourishment. These transformations may sound fantastical, but they'll become practically automatic as you change your body chemistry. Right now, your brain is exposed to unhealthy amounts of vegetable-oil-derived compounds. Once you start avoiding these fats and seeking out fats your appetite control center requires for normal function, you will begin the transformation.

THE BODY-MIND CONNECTION

If you've heard the expression "the mind-body connection," you probably know that our thoughts, feelings, beliefs, and attitudes can positively or negatively affect our biological function. For example, emotions like anxiety can trigger adrenaline release, which elevates our heart rate and makes us sweat. Bad news or difficult relationships can make us depressed, reducing the feel-good chemicals in our brain in ways that make us tired and physically impact our ability to perform in school, at work, and at home.

But I believe we're also driven by the reverse, the *body-mind* connection. In fact, I believe this body-mind connection is the far more powerful factor influencing our behavior and our health. After all, we are built of chemicals—not just our body but also our brain. Our brain responds automatically to chemicals just as nature programmed it to do. What I'm suggesting might sound extreme, but the balance of biological evidence suggests that we humans, as complex and amazing as we may be, are no more in control of our brains' reaction to certain chemicals than a single-celled organism is.

In fact, the chemicals driving our behavior are also present in bacteria, and drive the bacterial equivalent of a number of human behaviors. For example, our brain produces serotonin, a neurotransmitter that our brain cells use to communicate. Serotonin increases our desire to be social, and increases our interest in the opposite sex. The very same serotonin molecule affects bacteria in an analogous way. Serotonin induces cell aggregation in *Escherichia coli* on a petri plate, enabling single-celled bacteria scattered across the culture medium to come in contact with each other and share genetic material. Beyond driving bacteria to "socialize," serotonin also facilitates reproduction, and the absence of serotonin inhibits it.[5]

Of course, we are much more complex than bacteria. You can't simply spray serotonin on two warring countries and create peace and harmony, although that would be nice.

Very much unlike a colony of single-celled bacteria, we can be made aware of our behaviors and come to understand how chemicals may be influencing them. That's exactly what I hope this chapter will do. You will learn to understand how abnormal body chemistry may be influencing your moods, your behavior, your appetites, and the choices you make every single day. And you'll learn what to expect as your metabolic recovery enables your appetite control systems to operate properly again.

---

5 A. Oleskin et al., "Effect of Serotonin (5-Hydroxytriptamine) on the Growth and Differentiation of Microorganisms" [in Russian], Mikrobiologiia 67, no. 3 (1998): 305–312.

If you know anyone who went on a diet, lost weight successfully, and has kept it off for years, they owe this success to the part of their brain that regulates appetite. I've worked with plenty of people whose husbands or wives or sisters or brothers went through the very same program they did and were baffled as to why their weight loss partner lost more weight or kept the weight off longer. It's not that the successful person has a faster metabolism. It's that the part of their brain that controls their cravings was operating with greater efficiency.

The Fatburn Fix Plan gets you away from the fats that damage your brain's appetite control center, an absolute requirement for lasting weight loss that has been completely overlooked.

THE SCIENCE OF HUNGER

You may think your hunger and food cravings come from your stomach. But in reality they're coming from your entire body. The many signals your body's tissues generate regarding their respective needs for energy and nutrients are collected and interpreted by a tiny part of your brain called the *hypothalamus*. The hypothalamus then sends impulses to your cortex where they can be translated to your awareness. If your hypothalamus determines that you need to eat, then it sends signals to your cortex that makes you think about food. This network is operational 24/7, including while you're eating. If you are in the middle of a meal but your hypothalamus determines you should stop eating before you're done, you stop—unless you feel it would be impolite. If you don't stop, you at least pause to consider whether you want to clean your plate or not. If you end up overeating, say because your parents trained you to clear your plate from an early age, then the next day your slightly overstuffed body fat responds. It signals to the hypothalamus you have energy to burn, and your hypothalamus responds by dialing up your energy, thus increasing activity and calorie burn. This is how a healthy hypothalamus prevents a moment on the lips from becoming a lifetime on the hips. Or, rather, this is how it's all *supposed* to go down.

The ability to build and maintain a lean and healthy physique is a fundamental body function. Like breathing and having a pulse, our body composition is not supposed to be something we have to stress about. The rule holds even as we grow older, because healthy aging reflects a lesser need for strength (due to accumulated wisdom, in theory), manifesting as a body composition with a little less of *everything*—muscle, bone, and fat.

If you've experienced increasing difficulty sustaining weight loss, it's not that you need more willpower, and it's not an inevitable part of aging. It's because a part of your brain is inflamed and no longer able to serve its primary function.

HOW HUNGER AND FULLNESS MAKE YOU STRONGER

Your brain is in charge of regulating what you eat, when you eat, and how much you eat. It's where our food cravings, hunger, and sense of fullness register in our consciousness. The hypothalamus sits at the base of the brain directly between the eyeballs, behind the bridge of the nose.

When your hypothalamus is fully functional, body-weight regulation is automatic. You aren't obsessed with snacks or desserts because you crave healthy foods. You only get really hungry when your body needs nutrition. If you occasionally overeat and thus increase your body fat by a fraction of a percentage, your activity increases, your desire to eat declines, and your body composition ends up exactly where you started. All of this should happen without using your scale or apps for tracking what you eat because a healthy hypothalamus does all the calculating for you.

This automatic body-weight-regulating system relies on a myriad of hormones and other signaling molecules that act like dipsticks, telling your brain at what level your body's various nutrient stores sit at any given moment. When the stores are full, your tissues produce more of their "I've got what I need" compound. These signaling compounds make their way to the hypothalamus, which interprets them all and dials up or down your hunger and your activity and even directs your cravings for specific flavors, textures, and dishes.

Your hypothalamus dials up your hunger for days at a time after, for example, you participate in one of those Tough Mudder events that involves several long hours of running, climbing, and calisthenics. After all that exercise, your muscles generate *myokines,* special hormones that signal to your brain that they're going to do some rebuilding and could use a shipment—or two, or three—of raw materials. On receiving the myokine signal, your hypothalamus should dial in cravings for savory and salty flavors that, in an MSG-free world limited to real food, reliably guide you to high-protein and mineral-rich foods your body needs. These raw materials enable the exercise you did to stimulate new growth of stronger muscle. The myokines may also make you feel a little sore, maybe even more tired for a little while, which helps you rest your body so it can carry out the complex task of making you stronger, better, and faster, boosting your performance in the next athletic challenge.

On the other hand, if you just ate a big holiday dinner with a lot of cake and ice cream, then your body fat generates its "fat and happy" signal in the form of the hormone *leptin*. When that signal reaches your hypothalamus, it boosts your energy the next day so that you can burn off the excess. This explains why some people think they can eat more than other people. It's not that their metabolism is faster; it's that their appetite control systems dial up activity so that they simply burn it all off.

An article published in *Science* in January 1999 highlights the role of appetite control systems in maintaining normal weight. Researchers at the Mayo Clinic fed study volunteers 1000 extra calories per day for eight weeks and measured participants' activity levels and weight. On one extreme was a person who spontaneously increased their activity to the point where they burned all 1000 additional calories each day, and avoided gaining weight during the entire eight weeks. On the other extreme was a person who reduced their activity, burning 300 fewer calories on average and put on a pound of fat every week.

This kind of research tells us that when our appetite control systems are functioning normally, it's not guilt that gets us up and moving. It's our body fat sending signals to our brain that we've literally got extra energy to burn by generating internal cues that make getting up and moving feel better than sitting—kind of like being a kid again.[6]

Leptin is just one example of a hormone that helps your brain regulate your body composition for you. Leptin's specialty is telling your brain how

6 J. A. Levine et al., "Role of Nonexercise Activity Thermogenesis in Resistance to Fat Gain in Humans," *Science* 283 (1999): 212-214.

much energy you have in your body fat. I already mentioned myokines, produced by your muscle in order to help regulate your protein intake. Other compounds produced by organs such as your bones, your gallbladder, and your intestine serve to inform your brain about your status of protein, minerals, fatty acids, and other nutrients. When your body is functioning as nature intended, you won't need a Fitbit or a calorie counter or a spreadsheet of your macros because the appetite control system measures all variables with greater precision than any technology, and responds to all variables reflexively by dialing your hunger up or down, modulating your cravings, and dialing back or boosting your energy.

Unfortunately, most people today are unable to properly modulate their activity level to meet their calorie needs. Nor can they properly regulate their calorie intake—or enjoy the satiation from truly nourishing foods. This makes weight gain inevitable and sustaining any weight loss nearly impossible.

What might cause this array of signals to fail, making you feel like your hunger rarely ceases and your satiety rarely sustains? The answer is vegetable oil.

Recent research reveals how living on vegetable oils—as we now do—has turned us into a nation of rarely sated, chronically hungry junk food seekers. The science of how vegetable oil makes us hungry can be divided into two fronts: first, how it activates hunger and, second, how it interferes with satiety. Vegetable oil makes us hungry by switching on the same kind of powerful hunger signals that smoking marijuana generates. And it interferes with satiety signals by driving up brain inflammation.

HOW VEGETABLE OIL TOTALLY GIVES YOU THE MUNCHIES, DUDE

A 2012 article published in the journal *Obesity* starts out with the assertion that recovering from obesity requires calming overactivity observed in the endocannabinoid system of obese experimental animals.[7] Endocannabi-

---

7 Anita R. Alvheim et al., "Dietary Linoleic Acid Elevates Endogenous 2-AG and Anandamide and Induces Obesity," *Obesity* (Silver Spring) 20, no. 10 (2012): 1984–1994.

noids got their name from cannabis—the botanical name for members of the hemp species—after scientists discovered that smoking weed gives us the munchies because compounds in marijuana can bind to and activate receptors in the hypothalamus that drive hunger. Those hunger-promoting receptors were named after the compounds that bind them: cannabinoids. The prefix "endo-" simply means "generated internally." Put the two together and you get the term "endocannabinoids."

Once this was understood, the question researchers asked next about overactive hunger was "Where does all the overactivity in the endocannabinoid system of obese animals (and people) come from?"

A great deal of the endocannabinoid overactivity appears to come from vegetable oil. Vegetable oil is high in linoleic acid, a PUFA we've talked about before. Linoleic acid is a precursor to several kinds of molecules that directly activate these hunger centers of the brain. In other words, linoleic acid can make us hungry very much the same way that marijuana gives us the munchies. Remember how we learned in the last chapter that our body fat has ten to twenty times the linoleic acid concentration of body fat from a hundred years ago (before the explosion of vegetable oil production)? This latest research represents a smoking gun directly linking linoleic acid in our body fat to overactive hunger.[8]

Remember how we learned in Chapter 4 (Meet Your Metabolism) that linoleic acid shuts down energy production? Considering what we learned in Chapter 4 along with what we just saw in this chapter, we can conclude that as long as a person's body fat is abnormally high in linoleic acid, then between meals and whenever else they might start to burn body fat, instead of providing energy, their body fat provides a powerful case of the munchies.[9]

---

8 Alvheim et al., "Dietary Linoleic Acid Elevates Endogenous 2-AG," Obesity.

9 Anita R. Alvheim et al., "Dietary Linoleic Acid Elevates the Endocannabinoids 2-AG and Anandamide and Promotes Weight Gain in Mice Fed a Low Fat Diet," Lipids 49, no. 1 (2014): 59–69.
Shaan S. Naughton, "The Acute Effect of Oleic-or Linoleic Acid-Containing Meals on Appetite and Metabolic Markers; A Pilot Study in Overweight or Obese Individuals," Nutrients 10, no. 10 (2018): 1376–1390.

HOW VEGETABLE OIL MAKES YOUR BODY FAT
INVISIBLE—TO YOUR BRAIN

The second way vegetable oil promotes hunger has to do with driving up inflammation that suppresses the feeling of satiety. The human brain is largely composed of the most highly unsaturated, highly unstable fatty acids that are particularly susceptible to inflammation. That means that your brain and its delicate appetite control system is particularly vulnerable to inflammation.

Inflammation in your hypothalamus makes it impossible for your appetite control system to function normally. Most of the signals generated by your body drive satiety, the sense of fullness, rather than hunger. So when inflammation cuts off the communication lines between your tissues and your brain, the default signal is hunger.

One of the most well-studied examples of inflammation jamming satiety signals is the leptin system. Leptin is a hormone that body fat makes in spades when your body fat stores are full of healthy body fat. Only when you lose significant body fat, down to single digits, will leptin levels drop.

Leptin is produced by fat cells when they are fat and happy. When they're skinny and hungry, leptin levels decline. This means the more body fat you have, the higher your leptin levels. And it means that when you lose weight, your leptin levels drop.

The leptin system keeps your brain updated on the status of your energy stores. When energy stores are full, lots of leptin travels through the bloodstream to your brain, where the high concentration activates a network of energizing nerves called the *sympathetic nervous system*. As long as your leptin response system is working, your body fat stimulates you to get up and be more active, burning off fat and thus maintaining a healthy weight.

The system breaks down when inflammation interferes with leptin signals. When your brain doesn't get the leptin signal, it has no way to know that you've got plenty of fat in your body fat stores. You can see your body fat in the mirror, but your brain doesn't know it's there. This is why many people with stubborn weight that just won't budge feel crazy hungry or tired after just a little weight loss. The body fat is still screaming, "We're all filled up," but not as loudly as it once was, and the drop in leptin signaling can trigger a kind of panic mode; your appetite systems are convinced you are starving—making you tired, hungry, prone to snacking and overeating at meals, and ultimately making you reverse your hard-won weight loss.

Leptin's energizing effect forces those with healthy metabolisms to move their bodies, to pull away from their computer screens, to put down their phones and get up and get busy, burning more calories after, say, a holiday binge. When your metabolism is healthy, you can partake in normal social celebrations while maintaining your normal weight—this is how our body is supposed to function. We eat too much on any given day, the next day we have so much energy we spontaneously burn it off. We eat too little, we get hungry for missing nutrition and actually crave nutrients, not calories, and so we seek out the kinds of healthy foods that generate satiety signals.

CRAVING NUTRIENTS VERSUS CRAVING CALORIES

Autism researchers have discovered a connection between brain inflammation and sensory overload that helps us understand the role of vegetable oil in limiting our ability to enjoy healthy foods when they're presented to us. It's been understood for some time that autism is associated with brain inflammation, and that when this inflammation affects the hypothalamic appetite control centers, our taste perception is distorted, leading to food aversions, finicky eating, and preference for sweet over more complex flavor profiles.[10]

The same kind of inflammatory processes may be at work in non-autistic folks simply because, as we saw earlier, vegetable oil promotes hypothalamic inflammation. This is why many of the folks I work with don't enjoy the more pungent flavors of fresh vegetables, fish, herbs and spices, and so on. When you crave sweet and starchy foods, what you're craving is calories, not nutrition.

Taste aversions may occur because an inflamed hypothalamus is not functioning properly and can only process the relatively simple flavors of blander-tasting foods, driving a preference for processed foods like

---

10 A. Aubert and R. Dantzer, "The Taste of Sickness: Lipopolysaccharide-Induced Finickiness in Rats," Physiology & Behavior 84, no. 3 (2005): 437–444.

crackers, pasta, and chicken fingers, severely limiting a person's food options so that it can be very difficult to follow a healthy balanced diet for very long.

In a sense, inflammation forces your hypothalamus to make you seek out the least nutritious foods in an attempt to at least "understand" whatever it is you're eating.

For as long as you've had vegetable oil driving inflammation in your hypothalamus, your ability to enjoy food has been distorted. For some, this translates to finding comfort in sweets and starches. For others, this translates to an inability to enjoy the more subtle savory flavors of whole, high-protein foods and seeking them instead from Doritos, chicken nuggets, cheese crackers, and other junk foods. Food scientists have tricked your brain into believing these junk foods are extraordinary sources of protein when in reality they're mostly MSG-encrusted starch.

SEEK FATS THAT ACT LIKE NATURAL APPETITE SUPPRESSANTS

The most satiating foods are those high in both cholesterol and energizing saturated and monounsaturated fats. This is why most people can't eat much more than three or four eggs—which amounts to less than 240 calories—before feeling we've had enough. Meanwhile, fats like those in vegetable oils are not energizing and are easy to eat too much of because they don't send satiety signals as strongly. This is why we can eat a thousand calories of French fries without batting an eyelash.

WHAT'S THE SOLUTION?

Cut your vegetable oil consumption so the inflammation can subside and your brain can recover. Your appetite control center will "unlearn" the unhealthy associations between junk food and energy and "relearn" how to help you crave real nutrition. Quieting inflammation in the appetite control center of your brain is an essential step required to keep weight off in the long term.

It takes time to rebuild your brain with healthy fats, and so any weight loss programs that don't account for the need to heal your appetite control systems set you up for regaining lost weight. In theory, rebuilding brain tissue takes years, but in practice my patients tell me that after just a few months they've already noticed a significant improvement in their tastes, cravings, and energy levels.

I want you to understand how inflammation may be affecting your relationship with food so you can turn your primary focus away from calories or weight and shift your mind-set to the more immediate goal of eliminating overactive hunger. Weight loss will be so much easier once the overactive hunger we discussed in Chapter 2 (The Hunger Games) is eliminated. And sustained weight loss will be so much easier once the inflammation in your appetite control center is gone. Once that inflammation is gone, you will actually crave healthy foods and *only* healthy foods—or at least mostly healthy foods. This is the holy grail of lasting weight loss because it prevents you from feeling deprived, giving in to impulses, and returning to old habits.

Maintaining ideal weight can be effortless—once you fix your fatburn and get healthy. If you give your body time to rebuild damaged mitochondria, regain hormone sensitivity, flush out toxins from your body fat, and calm the inflammation in the appetite center of your brain, you will be rewarded with weight loss that lasts.

SCIENCE BOX: HOW VEGETABLE OILS INFLAME YOUR APPETITE CONTROL CENTER

Scientists have long suspected that dietary fat disrupted appetite by causing inflammation.[11] At first the suspected culprit was assumed to be saturated fat. But more sophisticated experiments have proved that assumption wrong.

---

11 Seth S. Martin et al., "Leptin Resistance: A Possible Interface of Inflammation and Metabolism in Obesity-Related Cardiovascular Disease," *Journal of the American College of Cardiology* 52, no. 15 (2008): 1201–1210.

When scientists wanted to probe deeper into the origin of inflammation, they started by feeding people a meal composed of a mixture of fatty acids similar to a typical high-vegetable-oil diet, relatively high in polyunsaturated and low in saturated fatty acids. A few hours later, they removed some blood, and isolated out the triglyceride-rich lipoproteins containing fat from the study meal. Then they added special enzymes and a tiny section of blood vessels to stimulate the process of unloading fat from those FedEx delivery vehicles, called lipoproteins. At this point, they noticed the unstable fatty acids were being damaged by the enzyme in charge of moving them off the truck. In other words, they're fragile and easily damaged by transport.

When molecules break down this way, they cause the dangerous reactions called free radical cascades. This is an extremely pro-inflammatory situation, and not surprisingly they found a variety of inflammatory changes taking place: "The FFA fractions elicited pro-inflammatory responses inducing TNF and intracellular adhesion molecule expression and reactive oxygen species (ROS) production."[12] What this says is that molecular "noise" essentially blocks all the hunger and satiety signals sent by each of our body tissues, thus disrupting the network of communication between body and brain that supports proper appetite regulation.

THERE'S NO SUCH THING AS A HEALTHY SNACK

We get messages all day that try to convince us snacking is good for us. There are millions of web pages devoted to healthy snacking and a news article nearly daily on the latest healthy snack craze. Don't believe the hype.

Whenever you snack, you are teaching your metabolism unhealthy habits. Whether we're talking about snacking on candy or soda, fruit or

---

12 L. Wang et al., "Triglyceride-Rich Lipoprotein Lipolysis Releases Neutral and Oxidized FFAs That Induce Endothelial Cell Inflammation," *Journal of Lipid Research* 50, no. 2 (2009): 204–213.

nuts, protein bars or protein shakes, if you want to lose weight, you need to break the snacking habit.

When you snack frequently, the circadian clock in your stomach is set to alarm at whatever time you normally snack, and when that clock goes off, you get hungry. In other words, snacking trains your metabolism to make you want more snacks. The more times you eat on any given day, the more time you'll spend building fat instead of burning it. Just like anything else you practice, by snacking, you'll get better and better at building fat; meanwhile your metabolism almost never gets to practice burning it.

We can be tricked into thinking snacking is healthy if snacking makes us feel temporarily better. If we're tired and snacks give us more energy, we can easily be tricked into thinking that snacking is boosting our metabolism.

But don't be fooled. Even snacks that boost your energy are disrupting your fatburn.

THE ROLE OF SUGAR

So far I've focused mostly on vegetable oil, but no conversation about appetite regulation would be complete without considering the world's number one most habit-forming compound. You know the saying it takes two to tango? When it comes to appetite disruption, vegetable oil doesn't dance alone. It finds its soul mate in sugar, sweet and addicting, making it the perfect companion for an entity intent on destroying health.

As is the case with vegetable oil, sugar and blood-sugar-raising refined flours are nearly ubiquitous ingredients in processed foods. These two ingredients alone now constitute 66 percent of the average American's diet. It's like we're running a bizarre experiment on ourselves to discover what happens when you feed people vegetable oil and sugar and refined flours in as many meals as possible.

Many doctors, including myself, have written books condemning the overconsumption of sugar, and for good reason. As important as these arguments have been to the international nutrition conversations, to focus only on the carbohydrate element is dangerously myopic. The massive disruption of our appetite control systems comes not at the hand of carbs alone, but from a new set of metabolic vulnerabilities to sugar's harmful effects created by our ever-increasing consumption of vegetable oil. (See the figure on US diet and health, 1909–2000, in the Introduction.)

Please understand, vegetable oil is toxic to your appetite regulation systems even in the context of a low-sugar diet. But the combination of the two is what truly sets us up for appetite dysregulation, catapulting your metabolism into a cycle of hunger, weight gain, inflammation, and hormone resistance that is difficult to break.

The reason sugar needs a partner in crime is simple: we've been eating sugar for a long time. According to statistics, our carbohydrate consumption is about the same today as it was in 1900, when our rates of obesity were about a tenth of what they are now. And as shown in the following figure, while we've increased our sugar consumption over what it was at the turn of the last century by about 65 pounds per capita per year, we've

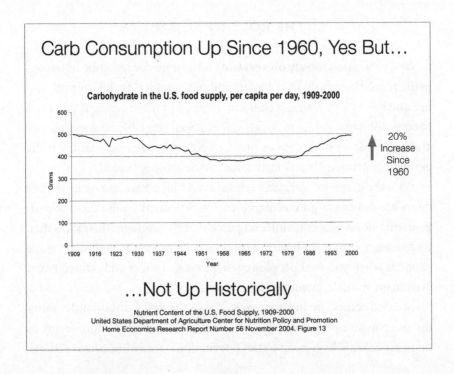

Carb Consumption Up Since 1960, Yes But...

Carbohydrate in the U.S. food supply, per capita per day, 1909-2000

20% Increase Since 1960

...Not Up Historically

Nutrient Content of the U.S. Food Supply, 1909-2000
United States Department of Agriculture Center for Nutrition Policy and Promotion
Home Economics Research Report Number 56 November 2004. Figure 13

decreased our consumption of flour quite a bit more, by about 100 pounds per capita per year.

Going further back in our history, humans have occasionally found themselves in circumstances where they needed to rely on fruits, tubers, and other sweets and starchy carbs for extended periods. So nature has developed a way of handling excess dietary sugar. As long as insulin and the other energy-balance hormones are still working as they should, then the human body can deal with occasional excessive sugar intake by quickly and efficiently removing it from the bloodstream before spikes allow sugar's sticky nature to cause troubles for our tissues.

A few hours after a high-carb meal, a healthy metabolism will be fueling with fat—thus staving off a snack attack and burning off fat you just built. A healthy metabolism may even make ketones on a high-carb diet because a healthy liver can readily convert body fat into ketones if we can go without eating for long enough.

A healthy metabolism can handle a certain amount of sugar for a long time, flipping quickly from using fat as an energy source to sugar and then back again to fat. This nimble fuel flip-flopping is called metabolic *flexibility*, and is one of the many feats an optimally functioning metabolism is capable of performing for you. So in my view, sugar should not be held responsible for today's massive obesity and chronic disease problem. For sugar's potential for harm to fully manifest, it must be combined with something that makes your metabolism less flexible and less capable of burning fat—something that makes you seek out ever increasing quantities of sugar.

As you read in Chapter 6 (Fatburn System 2: Hormones That Control Blood Sugar), refined carbs and sugar play a role in insulin resistance. But if you recall, I didn't say they *cause* insulin resistance; I said they *accelerate* insulin resistance. Leading obesity researchers consistently find that the most effective way to give an experimental animal insulin resistance is not by feeding it sugar, but by feeding it the vegetable oils highest in omega-3 and omega-6, polyunsaturated fatty acids, like soy, corn, and canola. When combined with a diet high in sugar and flours, the end result is excessive hunger, fatigue, overeating—and weight gain.

With all this damage continuing without being specifically addressed, it's little wonder that diets have failed you in the past. What's amazing is that you've been able to stick with a diet at all, which is testament to your willpower. Following the Fatburn Fix Plan will fix this fundamentally important problem of toxic body fat remaining behind after you've cleaned out your diet, and will enable you to use far less willpower and get far more satisfying results.

Now that you're familiar with the four fatburn systems and how they can be disrupted in any given person, you are ready to find out exactly where your metabolic health stands.

9

Fatburn Assessment Tools

No matter where I've practiced, from Tucson to Seattle to Hawaii to Napa to Florida, I have seen a consistent pattern of patients falling into one of three groups.

Those patients who are able to maintain their weight at or near what it was when they graduated high school into their retirement are buzzing with energy. They're unstoppable, filling every day with activities: gardening, cleaning, traveling, helping with the grandkids. They're living full and active lives, and when they come in for annual exams, they hop on and off my exam table like a teenager would.

By contrast, those patients who chronically struggle with weight quite obviously hesitate while considering how to navigate the climb on and off the table without getting hurt. These people are sometimes the very same people who talk about how in their younger years, back in high school or college, they were able to work hard and play hard. Nothing could hold them back. Keeping their weight where they wanted it to be was of no concern back then. It was practically automatic. But over the years, things changed. Now they find themselves strategizing to conserve energy every way they possibly can. They may only be in their forties or early fifties, but they're thinking like an invalid. If they go to an upstairs bedroom, they hesitate before heading back down the stairs. If the price tag of being overweight includes a reduced desire to move, you can start to see that people with weight to lose are trapped in a vicious cycle of weight gain, fatigue, fewer calories burned, and more weight gain.

A third group of patients sits between those two extremes. They don't quite burn fat optimally, but manage to sustain their energy by adopting a strategy of planning small snacks. Women frequently carry supplies of slightly sweetened drinks, candies, nuts, bars, and so on in their purse. Men frequently visit convenience stores, gas stations, and vending machines to get their energy fix. Many folks who adapt this snacking or grazing habit to maintain their energy can also maintain a normal or close to normal weight for many years, thanks to the fact that keeping energy up leads to more spontaneous activity, which helps to sustain their fatburn. These habits can keep them from falling into the weight gain trap, at least for as long as they can stay active.

Being able to determine your current fatburning ability is important to understanding where you should set your expectations for beginning the plan. Why not just dive right in to fasting or calorie restriction? What's wrong with losing four, six, or even eight pounds each week, week after week?

Some people can get away with it. People who have retained their ability to burn body fat can follow any calorie-restriction program, including fasting, and feel great the entire time. But the fact is *most* people with weight to lose are dealing with radically malfunctioning metabolism, and when they lose weight, they actually get worse at burning fat. As you learned in Chapter 1, losing weight without optimizing your fatburn first actually makes you a worse fatburner, setting you up to gain the weight back quickly and even overshoot, regaining more weight than you lost.

This chapter will help you use my clinically validated tools for assessing the health of your metabolism. The Fatburn System Assessment that follows assesses the function of each of your four fatburn systems. And there are also worksheets for assessment of snacking frequency, hypoglycemia frequency, and mealtime hunger frequency.

YOUR FATBURN QUOTIENT

The Fatburn System Assessment is a test that I've developed over the years for use with my patients. The test helps gauge the health of each of your body's four fatburn systems; the sum of the score of each of the four systems represents your overall Fatburn Quotient. The maximum score is 100; the minimum is 0.

Understanding how each of your body's four fatburn systems is currently functioning helps you to better appreciate that some of your health problems are related to your body's ability to produce energy, and will improve as you regain your metabolic health.

The lower the number, the less often your body generates energy from body fat and the more severely your body tissues suffer from inefficient energy production. As your numbers move up the scale, that tells me you are increasingly able to burn body fat. A Fatburn Quotient of 20 predicts your fatburn systems are functioning at 20 percent of their capacity. A Fatburn Quotient of 100 predicts that can you burn body fat with optimal, 100 percent efficiency.

The full quiz appears below. It is followed by a guided breakdown of each part of the quiz and each individual question, with further details on how to answer the questions and explanations on how those answers pertain to your metabolic health.

Part I: Mitochondrial Health

Q1: What is your resting pulse? Find your pulse in your neck and count beats for one minute. (If on blood pressure medications, circle 0.)

    <60 +7
    61–70 +5
    71–80 +3
    81–90 +1
    91+ +0

Q2: How often does this describe you? "The lower number on my blood pressure reading (diastolic) is usually below 80." (If on blood pressure medication, circle 0.)

    Almost always +6
    Occasionally or never +0

Q3: Does this describe you? "I have burning or uncomfortable sensations in my hands or feet and/or have been diagnosed with carpal tunnel or 'restless legs syndrome' and/or my hands shake when I am hungry or stressed."
  Yes +0
  No +6

Q4: Does this describe you? "I get headaches twice monthly or more."
  Yes +0
  No +6

Part II: Hormone Health

Q5: How often does this describe you? "I tend to get very tired in the afternoon between 3 and 5 p.m."
  Never +6
  Sometimes +3
  Frequently +0

Q6: How well does this describe you? "I have a really hard time losing weight, but I regain it rapidly."
  Not at all +6
  Somewhat +3
  Exactly +0

Q7: Does this describe you? "My fasting blood sugar is over 100, or my doctor told me I am prediabetic or diabetic."
  No +7
  Yes, my blood sugar is 100 or higher OR my doctor told me I am
      prediabetic +4
  Yes, I am diabetic +0

Q8: How often does this describe you? "My ankles and feet swell after I've sat for a while."
  Never +6
  Sometimes +3
  Often +0

Part III: Appetite Control

Q9: How often does this describe you? "I get heartburn or take medications to control heartburn (also known as GERD, gastritis, esophageal reflux)."
  I never or very rarely experience heartburn issues +6
  I experience heartburn once a week +3
  I experience heartburn twice a week or more +0

Q10: How well does this describe you? "I have a sweet tooth or crave starchy foods, and when they are around, I tend to eat more of them than I want to."
    Not at all +7
    Somewhat +3
    Exactly +0

Q11: How well does this describe you? "I tend to have something sweet or starchy at most meals, or I obsess about starchy and sweet foods when I can't have them."
    Not at all +6
    Somewhat +3
    Exactly +0

Q12: How well does this describe you? "I can lose a certain amount of weight, but then my energy crashes and I stop dieting."
    Not at all +6
    Somewhat +3
    Exactly +0

Part IV: Body Fat Toxicity

Q13: How well does this describe you? "I am the warm person in the room wanting to turn the thermostat down, or activity can make me feel uncomfortably hot or sweaty, especially when I'm pressed for time."
    Not at all +8
    Somewhat +4
    Exactly +0

Q14: How well does this describe you? "I take every shortcut I can—using the elevator and driving around the parking lot looking for the slot closest to the entrance."
    Not at all + 8
    Somewhat +4
    Exactly +0

Q15: How well does this describe you? "When I put on weight it tends to accumulate around my belly and neck or under my chin."
    Not at all +9
    Somewhat +5
    Exactly +0

SECTION A: FATBURN ASSESSMENT QUIZ

I recommend printing out several copies of the test so that you have blanks on hand to retest as needed. Some of the questions are self-explanatory, and explanation is provided below for the questions that require it.

This fifteen-question quiz assesses the health of each of your four fatburning systems: the energy-generating system (mitochondria), the energy-sensing and -regulating system (hormones), the brain's hunger system (appetite control), and the fat-storage system (body fat). How you answer each of the fifteen questions determines how many points you score on the quiz. In general, the higher your score, the better you currently burn fat and the sooner you will be ready to progress from one phase of the plan to the next.

As you take the quiz, you will come to understand that certain symptoms you may be experiencing may be related to your metabolic health and will therefore be expected to improve as your metabolic health improves. You can repeat this part of the test as you move through the plan to see how your metabolic health is improving, but it's not necessary. While your Fatburn Quotient predicts your current metabolic health and influences whether you spend weeks or months in Phase I, you need other information to know how long to stay in Phase I and when you are ready to progress to Phase II. That additional information is assessed by the tools in Section B of this chapter.

Part I: Mitochondrial Health

These questions assess the health of your cells' energy factories. While many diseases are now known to be a result of mitochondrial dysfunction, there has been no test that holistically assesses mitochondrial function—until now. This section will not only help you to assess the health of your most fundamental fatburn system; identifying the early symptoms of mitochondrial dysfunction will also help guide you to the actions I recommend you take (discussed in the plan) to improve the health of mitochondria in every organ before it's too late.

Q1: What is your resting pulse? Find your pulse in your neck and count beats for one minute. (If on blood pressure medications, circle 0.)

    <60 +7

    61–70 +5

    71–80 +3

    81–90 +1

    91+ +0

You can check your pulse by placing your fingertip over your carotid artery in your neck.

If you take medications for high blood pressure, you don't need to check your pulse and you will circle 0 on this question because many pressure medications reduce your pulse and therefore negate the value of the number. If you take blood pressure medications for something other than high blood pressure, for example to prevent migraine headaches, add 10 to your pulse and circle the number that corresponds to that sum.

Your pulse rate is driven upward by the sympathetic nervous system, which puts your body into fight-or-flight mode—both of which involve driving your heart rate up to pump more blood. When your body's mitochondria are dysfunctional, many tissues in the body are subject to energy fluctuations that, individually, activate the fight-or-flight response. When a significant portion of your mitochondria are chronically impaired, the fight-or-flight response is chronically elevated, resulting in a higher resting heart rate. The more tissues that are affected, the higher your resting pulse.

Q2: How often does this describe you? "The lower number on my blood pressure reading (diastolic) is usually below 80." (If on blood pressure medication, circle 0.)

    Almost always +6

    Occasionally or never +0

The official definition of "high blood pressure" has changed with nearly every one of the eight meetings held by the Joint Committee on Hypertension, but a diastolic pressure of 85 or higher is now universally agreed to be abnormal. Your diastolic blood pressure is the lower of the two numbers, and it represents how much pressure your brachial artery (the biggest artery in your forearm) sustains between heartbeats. You can get your blood pressure checked for free at any Walgreens in the country, as well as many other pharmacies and the YMCA. Machines at these locations are generally as accurate as those used in the doctor's office.

The science linking elevated diastolic blood pressure to mitochondrial dysfunction is the same as that linking it to increased pulse rate, described in the preceding question. Just as your pulse rate is driven upward by the sympathetic nervous system, so is your blood pressure, as both help push more blood through your heart and muscles in preparation for fighting or fleeing.

Q3: Does this describe you? "I have burning or uncomfortable sensations in my hands or feet and/or have been diagnosed with carpal tunnel or 'restless legs syndrome' and/or my hands shake when I am hungry or stressed."
    Yes +0
    No +6

I'm not referring to the "pins and needles" that commonly occur after spending too long in a position that places pressure on a nerve. I'm referring to other sensations that tend to occur in one or both hands or feet. While the "pins and needles" sensation is similar, the symptoms I'm referring to include burning pain or restless crawling feelings in the legs and are related to nerve injury due to more long-standing cellular damage.

Many people with tingling or pain in their hands who have been diagnosed with carpal tunnel but who do not have any associated weakness or loss of muscle are actually experiencing metabolic nerve injury in addition to pressure on the nerve from repetitive motion. Carpal tunnel, diabetic neuropathy, and restless legs syndrome are all now understood to be linked to damage to mitochondria in the nerves of the arms and legs, respectively. These symptoms can all improve with dietary changes.

Shaking is another indication of damage to mitochondria of your nervous system. While commonly blamed on too much caffeine, caffeine alone rarely causes hands to shake while your metabolism and the mitochondria in your nervous system are healthy. Another cause of shaking is a condition called essential tremor. If you have essential tremor, your hands shake at rest and they get worse with the added element of adrenaline. Parkinson's also causes hand shaking, although it's a very different kind of shaking—slower, more rhythmic, called "pill rolling"—and usually one hand is much worse than the other. All of these are now known to be symptoms of damaged and dysfunctional mitochondria in the nervous system.

Q4: Does this describe you? "I get headaches twice monthly or more."
Yes +0
No +6

Some headaches are due to normal hormone fluctuations associated with a woman's monthly period. But headaches more than twice a month indicate other factors. Although the brain tissue itself lacks pain sensors, the blood vessels that carry blood to the brain are highly sensitive to these kinds of stresses and are thought to be the source of headache pain, including migraines. Many headaches result when dysfunctional mitochondria fail to produce enough energy, and the energy drop can promote nerve swelling.

UNDERSTANDING YOUR MITOCHONDRIAL HEALTH SUBSCORE

The lower your score, the more serious the mitochondrial damage you're dealing with. When mitochondria are significantly damaged, not only are your cells resistant to burning fat and more dependent on sugar as an alternate fuel, but you also are exposed to dangerously high levels of inflammation that can generate serious impairments throughout your body, particularly the nervous and immune systems. Fortunately, given adequate nutrition and time, your mitochondria can recover, and even those serious neurological and autoimmune problems can improve dramatically. Reversing mitochondrial dysfunction takes time, so it's important to realize that the lower your mitochondrial score, the longer your sugar or carb cravings will stick around. Phase I focuses on learning foods that improve your mitochondrial health.

Part II: Hormone Health

The questions in this section are designed to assess the health of your energy-balancing hormones, particularly your sensitivity to insulin. It's vitally important to gauge your sensitivity to insulin because once you've lost normal insulin sensitivity, a small amount of sugar or carbohydrate can lead to very large spikes in your insulin level. Anyone with insulin resistance must strictly limit or entirely avoid the refined starches and sugars that deepen their metabolic damage. The lower your score, the more likely your arterial health is in need of the improvements that following the plan with bring.

Q5: How often does this describe you? "I tend to get very tired in the afternoon between 3 and 5 p.m."
   Never +6
   Sometimes +3
   Frequently +0

Afternoon fatigue is common due to the circadian cycle of cortisol, one of the hormones that the body designed to oppose the effects of insulin and to make us feel energized. Cortisol peaks early in the morning and drops by mid-to late afternoon, so it's normal to have a small dip in energy at that time of day. When your energy dip is disabling enough that you can't concentrate, however, that's an indication that your cortisol system is failing, likely due to being overpowered by chronically high insulin levels.

Q6: How well does this describe you? "I have a really hard time losing weight, but I regain it rapidly."
   Not at all +6
   Somewhat +3
   Exactly +0

This frustrating phenomenon is not your imagination. It's a reflection of the fact that your hormones have spent a lot of time being tooled for the purpose of growth of body fat, and this hormonal signature has dominated your metabolism for long enough that it becomes the default state.

It's a hormonal trap, and you've literally eaten yourself into it. The clean-burning fats and slow-digesting carbs you'll learn to use when you start the plan will help you to eat your way out.

Q7: Does this describe you? "My fasting blood sugar is over 100, or my doctor told me I am prediabetic or diabetic."

No +7

Yes, my blood sugar is 100 or higher OR my doctor told me I am prediabetic +4

Yes, I am diabetic +0

Your fasting blood sugar may be the single most important blood test you can get. If your fasting blood sugar is over 100, you've been a sugar burner for long enough to alter your body's glucose set point (see hypoglycemia discussion in Chapter 3). This is an indication that your body is resistant to insulin and possibly other hormones as well.

If you don't know your fasting blood glucose, you can call your doctor. Doctors almost always order fasting blood tests as part of a physical, and will almost always order glucose as one of the tests. If your blood sugar is just a little high, they don't, however, always tell you, so it's worth calling your doctor's office to find out the number yourself.

If you haven't had any blood tests done in the past year or so, I recommend paying a visit to get the tests performed. If you don't have a doctor, depending what state you live in, you may be able to purchase tests like this yourself directly from consumer lab sites such as DirectLabs.com.

Q8: How often does this describe you? "My ankles and feet swell after I've sat for a while."

Never +6

Sometimes +3

Often +0

I'm not talking about marks that show your sock pattern. I'm referring to a puffiness that makes it harder to see your ankle bones and the veins in your feet, which is more common in women. I'm also talking about edema, which is a condition that's more common in men and involves enough swelling that you see fluid collecting *above* a tight pair of socks. Both reflect the fact that insulin makes you retain fluid and salt, and chronically elevated insulin levels can cause puffiness or edema. This condition is called hyperinsulinemia, and it goes hand in hand with insulin resistance, as we learned in Chapter 3.

You can distinguish true edema from puffiness by pressing your finger into your lower leg. If the tissue indents and then leaves an indentation for a few seconds after you remove your thumb, that's edema. If it does not, that's puffiness.

Either way, the implication is the same: your body is overexposed to insulin and you are retaining both water and salt. If you have enough for your fingerprint to indent more than about an eighth of an inch, or your edema does not go away overnight, this is an indication that your metabolic issues have progressed from hyperinsulinemia and retaining fluid to kidney damage and possibly heart trouble as well.

UNDERSTANDING YOUR HORMONE HEALTH SCORE

Your Hormone Health Score is one way of assessing how far you've gone down the road of sugar dependence toward diabetes. The higher your score, the more likely you are diabetic or prediabetic. Determining whether you are diabetic or prediabetic requires simple blood testing, but either way the curative action you need to take is the same.

To correct this hormone imbalance, you need to do the opposite of what your body has been telling you to do. Your body has been telling you to eat frequently and consume lots of carbs, which is why low-carbohydrate diets, not medication, should be the primary mode of treatment for diabetes. You do not necessarily need to eliminate all carbs to derive significant benefit, at least not right away. Phase I will walk you through how much carb to eat and when you are ready to focus on hormonal healing with Phase I's Accelerated Plan.

SIGNS YOUR INSULIN HAS NORMALIZED

Since most people can't easily find out their insulin levels, it's helpful to know about the other indicators of improved sensitivity to insulin. Indicators of returning insulin sensitivity include:

- Fasting blood sugar levels returning to normal
- Triglyceride-to-HDL ratio of 2 or better, or lower than it was previously
- Increased frequency or regularity of monthly menstrual cycling or indicators of cycling (like headaches or moodiness)
- Reduced tendency to retain fluid or experience swelling with prolonged sitting
- Clearing or lightening of dark patches on the face or other sun-exposed areas
- Reduced tendency for allergies and minor infections, including yeast infection
- Thinning of any calluses that may have formed on the heels of your foot

The return of insulin sensitivity also often brings with it improved sex hormone function, which has important implications for family planning. I have had quite a few female patients conceive surprise children after going on low-carb diets. All had been told they were either infertile or too old, and therefore believed they couldn't have children and did not need to use any sort of birth control. I have also had several male patients experience doubling or tripling of their testosterone levels.

Part III: Appetite Control

Damage to the appetite control center manifests itself in two main ways: unhealthy cravings and hypoglycemia symptoms. Unhealthy cravings make you think obsessively about specific foods—usually junk foods your brain has become fixated on. These unhealthy cravings occur because your body fat is dysfunctional, tricking your appetite control center into thinking you are chronically underfed. As you learned, the appetite control center driving such irresistible food cravings resides in your brain and relies on information from your body fat and your gut. This system is extremely sensitive to damage induced by the two main ingredients in processed foods, which are the foods you will most likely reach for when your hunger is out of control.

Hypoglycemia symptoms, on the other hand, make you feel physically unwell, reflecting energy deficiencies anywhere in your nervous system that force you to stop what you're doing and seek energy immediately— even if it means eating foods you know are unhealthy. Hypoglycemia symptoms trick you into thinking you are eating less than you actually do eat. Hypoglycemia symptoms must be eliminated before your appetite centers can begin to heal, and you will eliminate them in Phase I of the plan. In Section B of this chapter you'll find a tool for assessing your hypoglycemia symptoms. The questions in this section of the Fatburn Quiz will assess overactive cravings occurring from inflammation in your body (your gut and body fat) that jams the signals your appetite control system needs to receive.

Q9: How often does this describe you? "I get heartburn or take medications to control heartburn (also known as GERD, gastritis, esophageal reflux)."
    I never or very rarely experience heartburn issues +6
    I experience heartburn once a week +3
    I experience heartburn twice a week or more +0

If you have been diagnosed with any of the above, or if you notice that spicy, acidic, or greasy foods upset your stomach in any way, this is likely a direct result of inflammation in your gut driven by vegetable oil and or a high intake of refined carbohydrates. Answer this based on your experience in the last few weeks. Some folks can control their heartburn by avoiding certain foods, so if you have been avoiding them and not experiencing heartburn in the past few weeks, answer accordingly.

Some people with gut inflammation develop ulcers; others develop autoimmune inflammatory diseases like Crohn's disease. When you eliminate vegetable oil and swap out refined carb for slow-digesting carb, your gut inflammation can begin to subside and even autoimmune disease can significantly improve. This gut recovery is essential for restoring normal appetite balance.

Q10: How well does this describe you? "I have a sweet tooth or crave starchy foods, and when they are around, I tend to eat more of them than I want to."

Not at all +7
Somewhat +3
Exactly +0

By "starchy foods," I mean bread (bagels, muffins, pancakes, waffles), oatmeal (even if not sweetened), or potatoes (i.e., hash browns). Starchy foods are simply sweets in disguise, as your body converts starches into sugar during the process of digestion. The more sugar you habitually eat, the more you need to eat in order to detect the same degree of sweetness. The more starch you eat, the more starchy food you need to eat before you feel satisfied. Both of these can promote the growth of unhealthy flora in the gut, and lead to inflammation.

Q11: How well does this describe you? "I tend to have something sweet or starchy at most meals, or I obsess about starchy and sweet foods when I can't have them."

Not at all +6
Somewhat +3
Exactly +0

Even if you don't crave them, if you actually eat sweets or starches frequently, you are likely disturbing gut and brain satiety. Sweets and starches feed unhealthy organisms in your gut that disrupt the gut's ability to produce satiety signals. And sweets in particular can also numb your sensitivity to the natural sweetness present in foods like nuts, seeds, and vegetables, depriving you of the pleasure you would otherwise feel when eating all kinds of healthy dishes.

Q12. How well does this describe you? "I can lose a certain amount of weight, but then my energy crashes and I stop dieting."
   Not at all +6
   Somewhat +3
   Exactly +0

If you've gone on any diet and successfully lost weight, but you've noticed that your energy was down as a result, this is a concern because it indicates that you may be experiencing fatigue due to abnormal leptin function (remember, leptin is a hunger-regulating hormone that signals to your brain that you have plenty of energy and can afford to be active). We've long known that leptin prevents hunger by acting on the central appetite-regulating centers in the brain. Scientists have very recently discovered that leptin deficiency also affects the entire body by depriving your nervous system of chemicals that your appetite control system normally releases to give you energy. When you have too little energy, it may be difficult for you to go out and exercise, and after you do so, your energy may crash for the rest of the day. Calming inflammation by cutting vegetable oils will improve your sensitivity to leptin, reduce your hunger, and increase your energy.

UNDERSTANDING YOUR APPETITE CONTROL SCORE

Scoring here works a little differently than the other sections. If you scored low on the sweet-craving question, then keep in mind that you will need to follow the "Extract Your Sweet Tooth" protocol (see page 229) during the Fatburn Fix Plan, regardless of how you answer the other questions in this section. If you scored low on the question about heartburn, you will benefit from the gut-healing pre- and probiotic foods. And if you scored low on the energy-crash-with-diet question, you would benefit from avoiding intense exercise more than once a week and focusing on light cardio activity.

Part IV: Body Fat Toxicity

These questions assess how much junk fat you have accumulated in your body fat. When cells try to burn this toxic fat, they may not be able to produce energy as efficiently as they should, and you develop the symptoms assessed in this section.

Q13: How well does this describe you? "I am the warm person in the room wanting to turn the thermostat down, or activity can make me feel uncomfortably hot or sweaty, especially when I'm pressed for time."
    Not at all +8
    Somewhat +4
    Exactly +0

If during the course of normal standing or seated work you often want to reduce the thermostat setting, take off your sweater, wear shorts to work, or wish you had a fan on your face when other people are comfortable (or cold), you should circle "somewhat" or "exactly" here according to how often the symptoms occur.

If you notice that activity like walking, stair climbing, or rushing through tasks or errands or appointments makes you feel uncomfortably warm, you should circle "somewhat" or "exactly" here according to how often the symptoms occur.

Q14: How well does this describe you? "I take every shortcut I can—using the elevator and driving around the parking lot looking for the slot closest to the entrance."
    Not at all + 8
    Somewhat +4
    Exactly +0

If you are regularly sleep-deprived, this may impact your answers to both of these questions and bring down your score in this section. That still provides meaningful information because being sleep-deprived makes changing habits much more difficult and can set you up for energy crashes in the afternoon or after exercise, as well as generalized poor concentration and reduced ability to learn. As you improve your fatburn, you blunt abnormal adrenaline and cortisol surges that can keep you up at night, and your sleep quality will improve.

Q15. How well does this describe you? "*When I put on weight it tends to accumulate around my belly and neck or under my chin.*"
Not at all +9
Somewhat +5
Exactly +0

Belly fat and neck fat suggest the presence of an unhealthy kind of fat deposit associated with insulin resistance, body fat stores having reached their limit, inflammation-prone fat cells, and fat building up in your arteries.

UNDERSTANDING YOUR BODY FAT SUBSCORE

The lower your score in this section, the more inflammatory your body fat and the less your body wants to burn it. The symptoms you develop, as identified by the questions in this section, are either direct or indirect results of cellular damage due to inflammation. Not only that, the more fat you do lose, the more damage your cells sustain. This toxic effect can make you subconsciously limit your activity and can even make you feel bad (tired or achy and uncomfortable) immediately after exercise or the next day. To escape this toxic body fat trap, you will need to replace the toxic fatty acids in your body fat with healthy ones. In the plan, you will find out what to eat to most rapidly detoxify your body of the junk fat that's making you sick.

UNDERSTANDING YOUR FATBURN FACTOR

SUGAR BURNER		FATBURNER	
High Risk	Needs Work	Above Average	Elite
0–25	26–50	51–75	76–100

SECTION B: SNACKING, HYPOGLYCEMIA, AND MEALTIME HUNGER ASSESSMENTS

This section provides tools that give you insights into how your hunger has been impacted by your metabolic health and how that in turn has impacted your habits. Tracking hunger symptoms and eating patterns will give you guidance on how your metabolic healing is progressing. This helps you know when you have improved enough from following the meal-planning ideas in Phase I and are ready to progress to Phase II.

The section has three parts. The first, the Snacking Frequency Assessment, quantifies how severely your eating habits have been warped by metabolic damage, blocking fatburn. The second, the Hypoglycemia Frequency Assessment, quantifies how often you experience energy emergencies that change your moods; these symptoms must be eliminated for you to succeed. The third, the Mealtime Hunger Frequency Assessment, quantifies how often you feel hungry between meals. This is essential to determining when you are ready to progress from Phase I to Phase II. It also helps you to distinguish hunger you can safely ignore from hunger you need to do something about.

SNACKING FREQUENCY ASSESSMENT

The funny thing about the human mind is that it is really good at tricking us into doing things without us really being aware of why. Sometimes it's only after you've been forced to document everything you put in your mouth that you recognize how much you were snacking.

The snacking frequency worksheet helps you tally how often you snack on a weekly basis.

The goal of this assessment is twofold. First, it will help you take inventory of how often you snack on a weekly basis. Second, when reviewed in combination with the Hypoglycemia Frequency Assessment, you can determine whether any snacking you do is driven by hypoglycemia.

SNACKING FREQUENCY

Place a mark in the box for every time frame you snack on a given day.
If you snack once in the AM, place one mark. If two, place two

	MON	TUE	WED	THU	FRI	SAT	SUN
MORNING							
AFTER-NOON							
EVENING							
Subtotal							
Weekly Total		Tally up the marks for each day in the Subtotal Row Tally up the marks for the entire week in the Weekly total row						

SNACKING FREQUENCY WORKSHEET

What Counts as a Snack?

Anything that you eat or drink that contains calories and is consumed an hour or more before or after your meal.

If you have a beverage like coffee in the morning at 6 a.m. and then have breakfast at 8, mark the 6 a.m. coffee as a morning snack.

If you have coffee with your breakfast, it does not count as a snack.

If you don't eat breakfast but you drink coffee, that coffee is actually your breakfast.

A Tic Tac counts as a snack, and so do cough lozenges.

USING YOUR SNACKING FREQUENCY ASSESSMENT

Complete at least one weekly Snacking Frequency Assessment before you begin implementing any changes. This will give you your baseline snacking frequency. Whatever the number is when you start, as you begin Phase I, the goal is to get the weekly total lower and lower every week. Once it's down to 0 *and* you are not experiencing hypoglycemia symptoms, you are ready to progress to Phase I's Accelerated Plan.

HYPOGLYCEMIA FREQUENCY ASSESSMENT

A lot of my patients don't recognize how symptoms of hypoglycemia are actually driving them to eat. As with snacking, for some folks, only by documenting symptoms can they recognize how uncomfortable they've been feeling.

The hypoglycemia frequency worksheet will help you tally how often you experience hypoglycemia on a weekly basis.

The goal of this assessment is twofold. First, it will help you to take inventory of how often you experience hypoglycemia symptoms on a weekly basis. Second, when reviewed in combination with the snacking assessment, you can determine how hypoglycemia symptoms may have been causing you to snack.

Remember, hypoglycemia is not simply normal hunger. It refers to a set of eleven low blood sugar symptoms (see below), and it represents a metabolically abnormal hunger that occurs when your body's cells are deprived of energy they need. It's important to track how often you have hypoglycemia so you can be sure you are taking the right actions to reduce it.

HYPOGLYCEMIA FREQUENCY

Place a mark in the box for every time frame on the days you experience
any of the 11 hypoglycemia symptoms

	MON	TUE	WED	THU	FRI	SAT	SUN
MORNING							
AFTER-NOON							
EVENING							
Subtotal							
Weekly Total		Tally up the marks for each day in the Subtotal Row Tally up the marks for the entire week in the Weekly total row					

HYPOGLYCEMIA FREQUENCY WORKSHEET

What Counts as a Hypoglycemia Symptom?

Any of the following symptoms that are present when you are hungry and that go away when you eat something. If they do not go away with eating, they may be due to another cause and do not count as hypoglycemia. (Please note: if any of these are recurring symptoms, you should discuss them with your doctor to secure a solid diagnosis.)

1. Anxiety
2. Brain fog
3. Dizziness
4. Fatigue
5. Heart palpitations
6. Headache
7. Irritability
8. Nausea
9. Shakiness
10. Sweats
11. Weakness

Because hypoglycemia symptoms are closely tied to your current state of fatburn, their disappearance serves as a reliable indicator that you have completed the first phase of your metabolic recovery.

USING YOUR WEEKLY HYPOGLYCEMIA FREQUENCY ASSESSMENT

Complete at least one weekly Snacking Frequency Assessment before you begin implementing any changes. This will give you your baseline hypoglycemia frequency. Whatever the number is when you start, as you begin Phase I, the goal is to get the weekly total lower and lower every week. Once it's down to 0 *and* you are not snacking, you are ready to progress to Phase I's Accelerated Plan. Because the Accelerated Plan is optional, you can elect to continue with the Baby Steps until you're ready for Phase II. You will use the Mealtime Hunger Frequency Assessment worksheet to make that determination.

MEALTIME HUNGER FREQUENCY ASSESSMENT

This worksheet helps to quantify how often you feel hungry at mealtimes. It's very important to assess mealtime hunger for two reasons. First, when you are hungry at meals, it can tend to make you put too much food on your plate—so you want to be aware. Second, and more important, is that once mealtime hunger is gone, it means you are ready to progress from the first metabolic rehabilitation phase to the second fatburn phase, where the focus is losing weight.

Mealtime hunger is different from hypoglycemia hunger because it is not associated with any of the eleven hypoglycemia symptoms. If you have hypoglycemia symptoms at mealtime, that should be logged on your hypoglycemia frequency worksheet.

MEALTIME HUNGER FREQUENCY

Place a mark in the box for every time frame on the days you experience hunger at the indicated mealtime

	MON	TUE	WED	THU	FRI	SAT	SUN
BREAKFAST							
LUNCH							
DINNER							
Subtotal							
Weekly Total		Tally up the marks for each day in the Subtotal Row Tally up the marks for the entire week in the Weekly total row					

MEALTIME HUNGER FREQUENCY WORKSHEET

What Counts as Mealtime Hunger?

Mealtime hunger is any sense of hunger at meals that is not associated with any of the eleven hypoglycemia symptoms. It's especially important to recognize because it tends to make you put more food on your plate than you would when not hungry.

USING THE WEEKLY MEALTIME HUNGER FREQUENCY ASSESSMENT

Unlike the other worksheets, which you will use before you start the program to perform a baseline assessment and thus track your progress, you only need to start tracking the presence or absence of hunger at mealtimes once you are no longer snacking. Once you have had no mealtime hunger for one to two weeks, you are ready to try your hand at Phase II.

Your stomach actually develops habits. It can keep track of time and has its own circadian clock. This is what enables cats and dogs to wake us up or give us "that look" at the same time every day. The function of your stomach clock is to help prepare your digestive system to receive food, by secreting acid and mucus and revving up other digestion-related activities. This kind of hunger, coming from your stomach anticipating that you will be sending it food, is not associated with weakness, fatigue, or any kind of bad feeling other than perhaps a slight tinge of mild nausea.

Feeling hungry before eating is actually a good thing when your appetite-regulating system is working and you are free of hypoglycemia. Pre-meal hunger helps you to enjoy what you're eating. Learning to interpret this hunger can help guide you to nutrients you might be needing—salts, protein, acid, antioxidants.

How to Progress Through the Plan

If your score on the Fatburn Assessment Quiz was 79 or less, then once you have had no mealtime hunger for one to two weeks, and you've been free of hypoglycemia symptoms during that time, you are ready to progress to the Phase I Accelerated Plan, where you focus on detoxifying your body fat rapidly using a keto or near-keto diet.

If you scored 80 or higher on your Fatburn Assessment Quiz, then once you've had no mealtime hunger for one to two weeks, and you've been free of hypoglycemia symptoms during that time, you may skip the Accelerated Plan and advance directly to Phase II, where you focus on losing weight by practicing intermittent fasting.

HOW DID YOU DO?

By now, you have gained a powerful understanding of your own metabolic health. And you can better appreciate the fact that being able to burn body fat is not about using willpower to fight off hunger and spending hours in the gym.

As you've been reading through these pages, you may have noticed that the Fatburn Fix Plan is as much about unlearning as it is about learning. That's because we've not appreciated the problem of weight gain in its full depth before proposing solutions. The upside of that sad legacy is that if you've followed other diets, your experience with this one should be significantly better.

You're going to be able to forget the idea that a healthy diet should be about deprivation, severe calorie restriction, and not having the rich foods that bring you pleasure. You can also forget the idea that you can force your metabolism into burning fat simply by depriving it of the calories your hunger constantly demands. But you'll also need to abandon the notion that slamming your body with a load of carbohydrates for breakfast is going to somehow turbocharge your metabolism to get you burning more calories all day.

The Fatburn Fix Plan operates under the not-so-radical proposition that when your metabolism is healthy, your desire for food will guide you to take in the number of calories your metabolic workload demands—no more, no less.

And this may be the toughest concept to unlearn: your body fat does not have to be your enemy. When your cells are healthy and your metabolism is healthy and your body fat is healthy, all your body systems will finally get the chance to conspire in your favor, to give you the happy relationship with food you may have never experienced before.

Now that you've established your current state of metabolic health, understand what your Fatburn Quotient tells you about your fatburn systems, and are familiar with how to use the Snacking, Hypoglycemia, and Mealtime Hunger Frequency worksheets, it's time to introduce you to all of the powerful metabolic healing tools you will learn to master as you progress through each phase of the Fatburn Fix Plan. If you want to discover the tools you can use to optimize your body composition and your health once and for all, you want to discover what's waiting for you in Part Three.

Part Three

THE FATBURN FIX PLAN

10

The Fatburn Fix Plan

How the Plan Works

IN THIS CHAPTER YOU'LL LEARN

- You will follow five rules from day one of the plan and continue indefinitely.
- Phase I prepares you for weight loss in Phase II.
- The best time to start a new exercise regimen.

HOW THE FATBURN FIX PLAN PROMOTES LASTING HEALTH

The Fatburn Fix Plan teaches you five rules that you will follow throughout the plan. The rules are guaranteed to bring about dramatic metabolic recovery and lasting health. The phases guide you through the creation of new dietary habits that will powerfully improve your health.

The Five Rules

The five rules of the Fatburn Fix Plan form the foundation of the plan. These dos and don'ts will hopefully become as natural to you as breathing.

1. Eat natural fats.
2. Eat slow-digesting carb.
3. Seek salt.
4. Drink plenty of water.
5. Supplement with vitamins and minerals.

In the next chapter, we will explore each of these rules in depth, which will give you an easy plan for what you should do (and shouldn't do) as you move through each phase of the Fatburn Fix Plan. The three chapters after that will teach you how to make fast easy meals that adhere to the five rules.

It's been my experience that lasting changes can only be made slowly, one step at a time.

That's why Chapter 12, the first of the three chapters describing the Fatburn Fix Plan, will teach you more basic skills using more familiar foods, and include tips for key habit changes that will make your transition to your new lifestyle as easy as possible. Chapter 13 teaches you how to take advantage of keto-style eating, and builds on the skills you learned previously. Chapter 14 teaches you how to use more advanced techniques like intermittent fasting and time-restricted eating.

The rest of this chapter will give you an overview of how the plan works.

THE UN-CRASH DIET

Doctors have tried to keep patients motivated by providing rapid weight loss. Today, most physicians who specialize in weight loss are essentially running medically supervised crash diet clinics. But according to national statistics, which show rates of obesity continuing to increase, this strategy has a dismal success rate. The problem is not a national motivation deficit. It's that rapid weight loss doesn't make sense, medically speaking.

You can't rush the development of a baby growing in the womb; a step-by-step orchestration of physiologic events must take place in the perfect order for a baby to grow. So don't expect any *Bring Your Baby to Full Term in Just Three Months* books, and don't hold your breath waiting for a drug to come along that promises to fast track your pregnancy. Babies are complex physiologic systems, and I hope you now appreciate that your metabolism is complex as well.

In order to rehabilitate your body's fatburning systems, we need to clear out the toxins from your fat stores, restore normal balance and receptivity to dozens of hormones, and calm the inflammation that disrupts your fat-distribution systems and distorts the way your nervous system perceives nutrition, energy balance, and flavor. Cutting calories right off the bat can force a damaged metabolism to burn toxic body fat, and risks deepening the hormone resistance problems.

That's why the Fatburn Fix Plan helps you to correct your metabolic problems before focusing on weight loss.

SET YOURSELF UP FOR SUCCESS

You may have followed a multiple-phase weight loss plan in the past. Most such plans start out with a rapid weight loss phase that requires extreme diet restriction and calorie deprivation. These dramatic habit changes rely heavily on your willpower. Those who are not healthy enough to fuel their cells with body fat often feel unwell and commonly fall off the diet in this early phase. Those who are metabolically able to burn body fat will move to the next phases of the plan based not on their physiologic state but rather based on whatever weight goal they choose. In each of the next phases, they are able to add back some more foods—and often end up returning to old habits, stalling weight loss or reversing it entirely. Your progress through the phases of these diets is not in any way tied to your physiologic state or metabolic recovery; the determining factor of when you move from one phase to the next is based on whatever weight goals you choose, and you are not given much if any guidance on how to determine those weight goals.

To my mind, a willpower-dependent, arbitrary goal-setting approach that does not give you the tools to assess your metabolic health and gauge when you're ready to burn fat makes less sense than a plan that matches your progress through each phase to your metabolic recovery and empowers

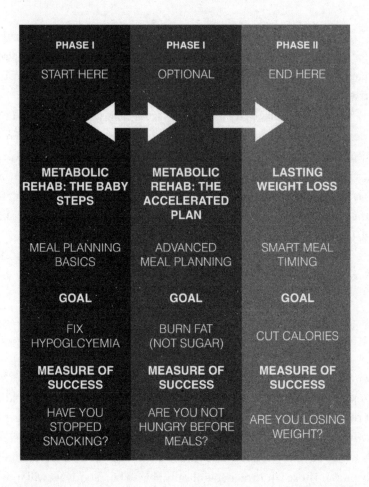

PHASE I	PHASE I	PHASE II
START HERE	OPTIONAL	END HERE
METABOLIC REHAB: THE BABY STEPS	**METABOLIC REHAB: THE ACCELERATED PLAN**	**LASTING WEIGHT LOSS**
MEAL PLANNING BASICS	ADVANCED MEAL PLANNING	SMART MEAL TIMING
GOAL	**GOAL**	**GOAL**
FIX HYPOGLCYEMIA	BURN FAT (NOT SUGAR)	CUT CALORIES
MEASURE OF SUCCESS	**MEASURE OF SUCCESS**	**MEASURE OF SUCCESS**
HAVE YOU STOPPED SNACKING?	ARE YOU NOT HUNGRY BEFORE MEALS?	ARE YOU LOSING WEIGHT?

you to make meaningful and sustainable habit change. That's why this plan works differently.

If you make too many changes at once, your body can rebel against you. You need to allow your body time to lay the groundwork that will set you up for lasting success. That's why Phase I is all about meeting you where you are and taking baby steps.

THE TWO-PHASE METABOLIC HEALING SEQUENCE

For you to succeed, the changes you make must be sustained. The Fatburn Fix Plan starts out by doing the preparation work that other diet plans skip. We start off by controlling your hunger and giving you more energy in Phase I. Once you've got more energy and your hunger is nearly eliminated, which you can gauge using the Hunger and Hypoglycemia Frequency Assessment worksheets, you're ready to focus on calorie cutting in Phase II.

Phase I

During Phase I you are ending the overactive hunger that drives you to snack or fall back into old habits. You need to control your hunger in order to stop relying on snacks to boost your energy and to be able to build new healthy habits that keep you away from junk food, fast food, and other sources of vegetable oils, starchy carbs, and sweets.

Your metabolic preparation work is an essential part of the goal of lasting weight loss. Phase I is broken into two chapters because, depending on your habits and your Fatburn Factor, you may need to spend more time taking the Baby Steps in Chapter 12 before progressing to the Accelerated Plan in Chapter 13. If your Fatburn Factor is 80 or higher, you can include meals from the Phase I Accelerated Plan right away. However, if your Fatburn Factor is 79 or less, then it's important for you to achieve total hunger-control for at least one to two weeks before moving on to the Accelerated Plan.

The Baby Steps chapter teaches you how to control the most common habits that you may have developed as your metabolism became more and more dependent on sugar. Habits like snacking multiple times a day, relying on treats to boost your energy, or indulging in a sweet tooth or frequent starchy cravings (drinking sweet-tasting beverages or relying on ready-to-eat food bars, takeout, drive-through, and microwave meals) are all working against you. If you have one or more of these habits, then I suggest you concentrate on the Baby Steps chapter until you've gotten both your hunger and these fatburn-harming habits under control. On the other hand, if you rarely snack, don't need treats to boost your energy, and already plan most of your meals at home or using whole food ingredients and a minimum of ready-to-eat and takeout, then once you've accomplished the goal of going one to two weeks without any mealtime hunger or hypoglycemia symptoms, you will be all set to take advantage of the Accelerated Plan.

Remember, once you have eliminated both snacks and hypoglycemia, you can jump back and forth between the Baby Steps and the Accelerated Plan as you please.

Even if you don't lose weight in Phase I, you are going to have more energy and fewer hypoglycemia symptoms. But most people find that their reduced hunger and improved energy naturally leads to weight loss from more activity and less sitting and eating.

Phase II

During Phase II, your focus shifts to weight loss. Thanks to the work done during Phase I, you will have improved your ability to use body fat for energy and can now safely cut calories without causing further stress to your metabolism. We cut your calories by restricting the number of meals you eat or narrowing the window of time in which you eat, taking advantage of both intermittent fasting and time-restricted eating techniques. You can accelerate your weight loss if you choose, either by increasing your physical activity or by fasting more often.

Now that your body fat is healthier, burning body fat actually energizes you, and you may notice you feel more and more energy the longer you go without eating. These metabolic improvements enable you to start to make the most important change of all, the one very few dieters actually achieve: restoring your body's ability to regulate your body composition.

THE ROLE OF EXERCISE

I've not emphasized exercise as a tool for metabolic recovery for a couple reasons. While lack of exercise definitely is not healthy, starting a new exercise program before you improve your metabolic health will be more difficult than it will be once you've become a better fatburner. However, if you already exercise, by all means please continue to do so because exercise has so many benefits. But if you don't yet have a habit of daily exercise, right now may not be the best time to start for two important reasons.

First, trying to start a new exercise program at the same time as you start the plan runs counter to the Baby Steps model. It's tough enough to consider all the new lists of foods, finding places to shop for the upgraded versions of some of your favorites, perhaps buying new containers, finding time to do a little prep work, and dealing with anyone else at home who may not be adapting to your changes. Heading to the gym in addition to all that may undermine your focus.

Second, exercise also tends to increase your appetite. This means there are timing considerations as well. For example, if you exercise before work but after breakfast, you may be so hungry after your workout that you're going to need a snack before lunch.

That said, once you have been following the plan long enough that you have more energy after work or after dinner or first thing in the morning, a regimen of light walking or easy videos or anything you enjoy is a great way to put that energy to use. In fact, as your energy improves, be ready to get tired of sitting on the couch for as long as you may have been used to. You need to be ready with something to do other than head back to the kitchen for food when you're not really even hungry.

A LITTLE WILLPOWER CAN GO A LONGER WAY

You know the saying "Work smarter, not harder"? This applies to exercise as well as to habit changes. The design of the plan is intended to make the most of your willpower, leveraging a little of that muscle to generate big changes to your habits. That's why the Baby Steps approach is so important. You need time to form new habits. It might begin as simply as including butter on your toast in the morning, thus energizing you all the way to lunch so you don't have to rely on a caffeinated beverage laden with unhealthy fats and sugar. This will allow you to drink more water. Each of these changes requires forming a new microhabit. For example, if you start using butter on your toast instead of jelly, you may need to buy more butter and you may want to keep some of it out of the fridge for easy spreading. Once you form new habits, it's no longer going to require willpower; you've set yourself on the right path and you can more easily keep coasting toward optimal health.

When we're talking about making hard changes and breaking undesirable habits, it's helpful to consider what motivates you in the first place. Do you want to look better? Feel better? Be able to put your children through college? Land a promotion? See your grandchildren graduate? Make better use of your retirement? There's no wrong answer, and you can have more than one motivation. But it's good to identify what motivates you so you can remind yourself of why you're doing what you're doing when the temptations arise.

One thing I've learned over the years is that the hardest part of making positive change is the part where you have to figure out if you actually want to make the change or not. Because once you decide you really do *want* to do something—when you're truly ready to commit—then you'll automatically start looking for ways that you *can* do it. And once you *believe* you can do something, you become unstoppable.

11

Five Rules That Fix Your Fatburn

IN THIS CHAPTER YOU'LL LEARN

- The five rules that fix your fatburn.
- How each of the five rules works.
- How to make following the five rules as easy as possible.

This chapter will introduce you to the five simple rules that fix your fatburn. Throughout the Fatburn Fix Plan's two phases, you will be following these five simple rules. These rules form the foundation of the plan. All by themselves the five rules are guaranteed to bring about dramatic metabolic recovery and lasting health. These dos and don'ts will hopefully become as natural to you as breathing. We'll start off by learning the most important rule of all.

RULE #1: AVOID VEGETABLE OIL

DO NOT Eat Vegetable Oils

This is my number one rule because it is THE most important rule: avoid vegetable oils as if your life depends on it. That's not always going to be easy;

if you eat like the majority of my patients, these oils compose one-third of your calorie intake and 80 percent of your fat calories. Unless you are purposefully avoiding them, chances are you are eating more than you realize.

I recommend you commit the six most common bad oils to memory: canola, corn, cottonseed, soy, sunflower, and safflower. There are three C and three S words to remember. The good fats and bad fats guide on page 341 (at the end of the Resources section) provides a quick reference you can photograph and use while shopping.

Many common food products contain these oils. Manufacturers add them to peanut butter since they are cheaper than peanuts. They add vegetable oils to pasta sauces, mayonnaise, and salad dressings instead of olive oil since they are cheaper than olive oil. Condiments, sauces, and dressings are especially tricky because on the front they will say they are made with olive oil, but when you turn the bottle around to read ingredients, you'll see soy or another vegetable oil listed first, meaning it's hardly got any olive oil. Other places where vegetable oils lurk include crackers, store-bought pastries and cookies, and chips of all kinds—even organic vegetable chips.

In other words, you need to look for them everywhere. It does not matter whether you are shopping at a 7-Eleven or a Whole Foods; these oils are in the store's products. To avoid them, you need to get in the habit of picking up every product and turning it around to read the ingredients list slowly and carefully. Even if the product is organic and GMO-free, these oils can be in there, so you need to look at the label. Even if the vegetable oil has been expeller-pressed, your health depends on your ability to avoid it.

To find products that do not have these oils, refer to the Healthy Shopping Guide tab on DrCate.com.

Bear in mind that it's perfectly OK to eat the foods that vegetable oils come from, like corn, soybeans, and sunflower seeds. When the oils are still in the seed, nature protects the fragile polyunsaturated fatty acids with antioxidants, vitamins, and minerals. The process of taking the oil from the seed is what causes these oils to become unhealthy.

This first rule is so important that if this were the only rule of all five that you followed, you would still be able to boost your fatburn. If you can get vegetable oils out of your diet and replace them with the healthy clean-burning fats nature intends us to eat, that one change alone will bring about dramatic improvements in your health and prolong your life.

DO Eat Natural Fats

One of the easiest things this program requires you to do is get more good fats into your life. Good fats come from animal fat and warm-weather plants like olive and avocado. They are high in the fatty acids we call *saturated* and *monounsaturated*. As you know from reading Chapter 5 (Fatburn System 1: Mitochondria), these fatty acids are stable, and unlike the bad oils, they do not break down in your body and do not cause inflammation. Because they are stable, they burn cleanly. This means your body can safely use them as fuel and they are an excellent source of cellular energy.

To make healthy meals as fast as possible, always keep your kitchen stocked with good fats, including olive oil, butter, peanut oil, and avocado oil. You can cook with all of these. Other good fats that you might really enjoy are bacon fat, coconut oil, and sesame oil.

All-natural fats have a lot of good flavor. In fact, the easiest way to know whether a fat is natural or a "good" fat is to think about what it tastes like. Do you know what canola oil and soy oil taste like? Pretty much nothing, right? Do you know what butter and olive oil taste like? Of course you do! They taste like butter and olive oil.

In addition to the oils themselves, you can save time by stocking your kitchen with a few staple prepared foods made with good oils. Mayo and pasta sauces are staple foods in many people's kitchens, so let's take a look at these two.

Most mayo contains unhealthy soy, sunflower, or canola oils. But you can find mayo made with avocado oil pretty easily. Chosen Foods, Sir Kensington's, and Primal Kitchen are available online and at chain grocery stores around the country. They do cost more than regular mayo, and some people notice a flavor difference in some brands but not in others.

Most pasta sauce contains unhealthy soy or canola oils. If you can make your own pasta sauce from scratch, that's fantastic. But if you ever need a short cut, Ragú makes a line using only olive oil and no junk oils that includes meatless and meat-containing versions. It's called Simply Chunky, and it's sold at many grocery stores—you can check local availability with this online tool:

www.ragu.com/our-sauces/ragu-simply/chunky-marinara-sauce

I'm not a fan of junk food, but when you need to bring a snack to a party or if you live with anyone who insists you keep junk food around, then you can buy junk food made with butter or healthy oils. For example, you can find cookies made with real butter, potato chips made with avocado or olive oil, and popcorn made with ghee or coconut oil.

Once you start looking for bad oils, you will find that they are in many foods you might not have otherwise guessed. Manufacturers love bad oils because they're cheap and have no flavor. That means they can use vegetable oils to essentially "water down" the main ingredient. Take a look at peanut butter, for example. You'll see most peanut butters have some kind of oil added, along with sugar. The natural peanut butter I recommend is made with just peanuts and salt. Yes, it will cost you more, but you are getting more peanuts for your money. Peanuts cost more than vegetable oils and sugar. So if you buy a product that has added oils and sugar, the reason it's cheaper is because of those unnecessary toxic fillers.

Now that you've learned a little about good fats and bad, you're ready for the next most important rule, which helps you pick out the good kinds of carbs and avoid the bad.

DON'T PANIC IF IT'S NOT ORGANIC

You may be worried you need to eat everything organic in order to avoid toxins that block your fatburn. However, the biggest factors blocking your fatburn have nothing to do with whether food is organic or not. Yes, organic can be healthier, and organic animal products are particularly likely to be healthier than their nonorganic counterparts. Pastured animal products are the best, so if you have a limited budget for organic, choose those first. Otherwise, do the best you can.

By optimizing body composition, the average person will reduce their food intake by 30 to 50 percent. That's going to be good for your bank account and your health. And if everyone was able to eat to match the needs of their ideal body weight, imagine what that would do to improve the future of the planet.

RULE #2: USE SLOW-DIGESTING CARBS

DO NOT Eat Sweets or Big Piles of Starchy Carbs

Now that you know how to sort out good fats from bad, you're ready to turn your focus to carbohydrates. Some carbohydrate-containing foods make you gain weight, while others can help you lose it. It's essential to learn the difference.

The two main categories of carbohydrates that you need to avoid are sweets and starchy carbs.

Sweets are easy to identify: they include most foods that taste really sweet, like cookies, brownies, cakes, muffins, candy, soda, and other sweet beverages. These foods are addicting and should not be eaten on a daily basis unless you are a fitness fanatic, and even then you should avoid them at breakfast when they are most addicting. If you have a habit of eating sweets, it can be difficult to break the habit, but the first step to breaking a bad habit is recognizing it's bad.

Sweets also includes most fruits and fruit juices. It doesn't matter that fruit has natural sugar. Sugar is sugar. The fruits we grow these days are so overloaded with sugar, they have relatively little else to offer in terms of nutrition. I'm not saying you can't eat any fruit, but fruit should be used more like a flavoring agent to make other foods taste better.

The fruits lowest in sugar are berries and melons. The fruits highest in sugar are dried fruits, like prunes, dates, and raisins. The size of the fruit also matters, and big fruits like bananas, mangos, and papayas have too much sugar to make eating the whole thing at one sitting a regular habit.

Starchy carbs include fluffy white foods like potatoes and rice and anything made out of mostly flour like pasta, bread, pastries, and crackers. These foods are full of calories and easy to overeat. In fact, many of us can't stop eating them once we get started. They are also nearly devoid of nutrition, which means that every calorie you consume has almost no value to your body and will serve mainly to make you build fat.

Still, it's nice to have these once in a while. If and when you do eat mashed potatoes, rice, pasta, or other starchy carbs, you may need to actually measure your portion sizes to prevent a starchy-carb overdose, at least in the beginning until you learn. More than 1 cup of rice or mashed potato per day is simply too much for a damaged metabolism. The less you eat, the faster your metabolism can recover. I recommend most people try their best to cut them out and eat the slow-digesting carbs instead, which you'll learn about soon.

DO EAT SLOW-DIGESTING CARBS

Slow-digesting carbs come from foods that contain some carb but won't spike your insulin in the way that your typical carb-rich foods can. Your digestive system breaks slow-digesting carbs down slowly, which makes these foods act kind of like a time-release sugar-delivery system. Slow-digesting carbs are generally found in whole or minimally processed foods.

A familiar source of slow-digesting carbs is vegetables. Almost anything you'd consider a vegetable is a good source of slow-digesting carbs. Common veggies include corn, broccoli, string beans, Brussels sprouts, beets, carrots, tomatoes, and asparagus, some of which have more carb than others. Other familiar sources of slow-digesting carbs are beans, like lima beans and kidney beans, nuts and seeds, like almonds and sunflower seeds, and intact grains, like wheat berries, sprouted wheat, and oat groats. Never heard of wheat berries and oat groats? These are simply the names for the intact form of wheat and oat, before they're milled or refined into flour or oatmeal. Never heard of sprouted wheat? This is wheat that's been partially germinated and can be mashed into a dough to make bread called sprouted grain bread that won't spike your insulin. Whole wheat *flour* is not a slow-digesting carb because the process of pulverizing grains into flour destroys the structure of the seed. It's the structure that makes slow-digesting carbs slow.

Slow-digesting carbs are basically whole foods that are encapsulated in nutrients that slow down the digestive process. These nutrients may be cellulose fiber, fat, protein, or some combination of all three. Cellulose fiber, fat, and protein slow digestion by getting in the way of the enzymes that break the starch into sugar. Slowing down the process of breaking starch into sugar means you're not going to get a big sugar spike. Instead, the sugar dribbles into your bloodstream slowly. That slow drip helps sustain your energy until your metabolism heals and you regain your ability to burn your body fat.

All slow-digesting carbs are more structurally complex than the starchy carbs, potatoes, rice, refined flours, sweet beverages, and most fruits.

One flour is an exception: nut flour. Nut flours are good sources of slow-digesting carb because even though the nuts have been pulverized, the fat and protein in the nut surrounds the starchy component, and thus slows the ability of your digestive enzymes to access the starch.

You'll be using slow-digesting carbs throughout the plan. These foods will give you more sustained energy than foods like cereal, fruit, flavored low-fat yogurt, pastry, muffins, or oatmeal. Slow-digesting carbs smooth your transition from a higher-carb to a lower-carb diet, allowing chronically high insulin levels to settle down during the Baby Steps portion of Phase I before you move on to the optional Accelerated Plan.

Time of Day Matters

You've probably heard it said that breakfast is the most important meal of the day and that if you don't eat breakfast, you're turning your metabolism to some kind of slow setting. This is based on the incorrect thinking that your metabolism is a simple mechanical engine that shuts down at night, so it needs you to "rev up the engines" in order to get started in the morning. The reality is your body does not shut down while you sleep, nor does it need to be "revved up" again in the morning.

I tell my patients instead that breakfast is the most important meal of the day not to screw up. Eating too much carb at breakfast does just that. The reason for this has to do with our daily hormonal cycles, particularly the morning cortisol pulse we read about in Chapter 6 (Fatburn System 2: Hormones That Control Blood Sugar). Thanks to these cycles, you can eat the same amount of carbohydrate at one time of day and it will have a dramatically different effect on your metabolism than if you eat it at another time of day. The worst time of day to eat carb is in the morning. If you want to eat anything sweet, or treat yourself to something starchy, the best time of day to do that is with or after your dinner.

Throughout the plan you can eat slow-digesting carbs. But I want you to always try to put off most of your carbohydrate intake until later in the day. We'll learn more about why this is better for you later in the plan.

RULE #3: SEEK SALT

DO NOT Believe the Claim That Salt Causes Health Problems

In medical school I heard salt take the blame for hypertension, arterial disease, and even cancer. Yet the evidence against salt is sketchy at best. Unbiased experts now warn that we've been blaming "the wrong white powder" because sugar is a much bigger contributing factor to chronic disease.

Due to the pervasive myth that salt is bad for us, many people don't add salt to their foods. Thousands are hospitalized every year with low sodium levels as a result. Many thousands more are walking around feeling dizzy, weak, and lethargic and misattributing it to age or even thyroid problems. Certain blood pressure medications and antidepressants increase the risk of developing low sodium. Such low sodium can make a person feel so awful that it's not uncommon for them to believe they are about to die. When you slowly and carefully give these people salt again, their blood pressure comes back up to normal and the improvements are so dramatic they seem to have bounced back from death's door.

If people have abnormally low blood pressure due to salt deprivation, giving them salt helps bring their pressure from too low back up to normal. But salt does not cause chronically elevated blood pressure.

The body maintains normal blood levels of salt, as well as vitamins, minerals, and many other key nutrients, through a process called *homeostatic regulation*. You don't need to know that term. You do need to know that it enables your body to take care of very important functions, like breathing, completely automatically. If I were to tell you that you need to watch the clock and be sure to take just eight breaths each minute because breathing faster than that exposes you to too much oxygen, I hope you wouldn't believe me. Well, just as nature manages how often you breathe by making you feel like breathing more if you aren't breathing enough, nature manages your blood pressure by making you want more salt if you're not eating enough.

A chronically low-salt diet makes it hard for your body to maintain normal function. For one thing, salt deprivation can reduce the kidneys' ability to eliminate nitrogen-containing by-products of protein metabolism. As the nitrogen wastes builds up, your kidneys try to dilute the toxic effects by retaining water, which can make your legs swell. Doctors often wrongly advise patients overloaded with toxic nitrogen and water to further reduce their salt intake. When this fails to improve the edema, we prescribe medications to force the kidneys to eliminate more salt, which helps with the edema but sometimes just for a few hours a day.

Many hundreds of thousands of people are walking around in such a state. When you throw in an infection like pneumonia or a complicated urinary tract infection to a person without enough salt for their body to function, this is a recipe for disaster and practically always requires hospitalization, usually in intensive care. Since most doctors are trained to believe salt causes hypertension, even though blood levels reveal salt deficiency, people are almost never told to eat more salt and often leave the hospital still low in total body salt and weakened by the infection. This often leaves them so enfeebled they can't care for themselves and are essentially ticking time bombs for repeated hospitalizations. Meanwhile, they will face a mountain of medical bills and debt.

The only time a person needs to deliberately track their salt intake is after one or more of their organs have failed and the body no longer achieves proper homeostatic regulation. Once this occurs, it's just as hard for the body to retain salt if the diet is low in salt as it is to eliminate it if the diet is too high. It also becomes necessary for these folks to carefully track their intake of potassium, phosphorus, water, and nitrogen as well as many other things that a healthy body does far more effectively on its own.

In summary, the wrong advice about salt causes incredible suffering every day. Fortunately, it's easily avoided if you are willing to follow this simple rule: seek salt.

DO Seek Salt

"Seek salt" is my favorite of all the five rules. It's easy to do. It's cheap. And it makes so many good foods taste so much better.

There are all kinds of salts you can buy: iodized salt, sea salt, Himalayan salt, Dead Sea salt, Celtic salt. What they all have in common is sodium and chloride minerals, the most essential components of table salt. Many of the specialty salts listed above have additional minerals besides sodium and chloride, such as magnesium or iodine. These specialty salts are wonderful, but they are also more expensive. I'll be recommending mineral supplements for those who can't get all the many kinds of salt required to help fill all your mineral needs.

Whatever brand of salt you have, adding more of it into your diet will help you burn body fat for seven different reasons that we will discuss.

Salt Reduces Hunger

Have you ever craved something salty? Since most of us associate salty food with snack foods, most people satisfy these cravings with foods they know are unhealthy, like potato chips, pretzels or crackers, French fries, stir-fry, or pizza.

Salt cravings are important warning signs that you may be low in salt. So it's important to listen to the craving. What it's telling you is that you need more salt. But most folks interpret these cravings as a need for food. This makes us overeat.

If you absolutely need to snack, choose something super salty but also healthy and low in calories, like a dill pickle, bone broth, or miso soup.

Salt Makes Healthy Food Taste Better

We've been so thoroughly brainwashed to believe that salt is unhealthy that now, ironically, the only time many people get any salt at all is when they're snacking on junk. By adding salt to healthy foods, you'll be making them taste better. Most people find that adding salt to their meals dramatically reduces the desire for junk food and makes it easy to enjoy larger portions of nutritious foods.

Salt may be the best-kept secret in the restaurant industry. If you've ever thought that restaurant food tastes better than food you make at home, it may not be a lack of cooking skill. It may be that you're working with the handicap of inadequate salt. Salt is instantly vivid; it brightens the flavor of just about everything. While you're not looking, chefs in all the best restaurants are pouring on the salt. "Correct seasoning to a chef is as much salt as you can put in without it tasting too salty," according to one celebrated chef. Author of *Cooked* and food guru Michael Pollan describes how, while cooking meat for a friend who is also a chef, he's instructed to "use at least three times as much as you think you should." Shocked, Pollan consulted another chef. He advised him to "up the factor to five."

Because the government recommends you limit your salt to unhealthy low intakes, it's not uncommon to get more salt in a single restaurant meal than the government recommends you get all day. This is one way that restaurant food is actually good for you. But don't expect the government to amend their error any time soon. Legislators in New York have already made one attempt to get salt banned in restaurants. According to *Time* magazine, federal legislation on salt content in restaurant food is under consideration.

Salt Helps Reverse Insulin Resistance and Diabetes

As we've discussed, insulin resistance is a huge obstacle to proper fatburn. Adding salt can actually help you to recover from insulin resistance and regain normal insulin sensitivity in your body.

According to Dr. James DiNicolantonio, an expert on salt and its benefits, chronic salt depletion may be a cause of a kind of internal starvation. When you restrict your salt intake on a regular basis, "the body eventually panics. One of the body's key defense mechanisms is to increase insulin levels," he writes in *The Salt Fix*. Insulin helps the kidneys hang on to what little salt remains. But insulin also shuts the door to the fat closet, preventing fat release between meals when you need it for energy. This makes your body burn up more of its sugar supplies and contributes to the problems of hypoglycemia and overactive hunger.

Salt Improves Your Digestion

One of the simplest home remedies for indigestion and acid reflux is sitting in your kitchen: salt. Salt gives your body two essential minerals, sodium and chloride. Your stomach needs chloride to make hydrochloric acid and your liver needs salt to make bile salts. If you add enough salt to your home-cooked meals, you provide both of these gut-function-assisting minerals. Taking a pinch or two of salt, dissolving it in your mouth, and then drinking a glass of water is reported to make upset stomach go away.

Salt Improves Learning and Concentration

You already learned that low sodium levels make people tired. The reason for this is that your brain requires normal salt balance to function. And when your blood sodium is low, your nervous system slows down. This can cause attention deficits, impaired memory, and balance problems. It can also trigger a killer headache.

Salt Improves Your Energy

If you start feeling tired and headachy at any time during the plan, eating salt usually helps quite a bit. You can usually prevent these feelings by making sure to consciously seek out salty foods with meals, like salted nuts or cheese, and add salt to foods like soup, salad, meats, veggies, and any other dish you desire. If you forget for any reason and find yourself with fatigue and headache, swigging a quarter teaspoon or so of salt, and washing it down with a few sips of water, will usually help perk you back up within twenty minutes.

Salt Improves Bone Health

As you already learned, when your diet is chronically low in salt, your body can experience a kind of internal starvation. The idea is that the body has to eat itself to feed itself—the ultimate borrow-from-Peter-to-pay-Paul scenario. One of the richest sources of sodium in your body is your bones. Studies show that low sodium levels force cells in the bone to start dissolving bone matrix in order to extract sodium for export into the bloodstream. Restoring salt balance by eating enough can easily prevent this.

How does improved bone health translate to accelerating fatburn and weight loss?

For one thing, a surprising number of people lose several inches of height as they age, women especially. Starting at around age forty, women lose an average of half an inch per decade. For men, height loss often starts after sixty. If you're in either category and have not checked your height in several years, you should. I've found a number of patients down two to three inches who had no idea.

Height loss matters to weight loss because the taller you are, the more calories you can eat without gaining weight. When it comes time to cut calories, the taller you are, the easier it is to cut calories while still eating three decent-sized meals and getting enough overall nutrition. Eating salt won't help you regain lost height, but it will help you stay at your current height.

How Much Salt Is Enough?

We are told to eat 2.3 grams per day, which is just over half a teaspoon. Optimal intake is actually between 5 and 10 grams per day, or 1⅓ teaspoons to 2⅔ teaspoons. You may need even more if you drink a lot of coffee, sweat a lot, or take medications that make you lose salt, like certain antidepressants or diuretics for blood pressure.

I don't expect you to add up all the salt you eat on a regular basis and keep track of it on a spreadsheet. But I do want you to make sure to consciously try to add salt to as many meals as possible.

There's almost no chance you'll get too much salt in your diet. Firstly, when you oversalt your food, it's pretty much inedible—most people spit it out. Secondly, 2⅔ teaspoons is really a lot of salt! Third, even if you exceed what you need, a healthy pair of kidneys will eliminate the extra.

Getting enough salt is also a great way to ensure you drink enough water. Which brings us to Rule #4.

SHOPPING FOR SALTS OF THE EARTH

There are two main categories of salt that you'll encounter, evaporated and mined. Evaporated salt can be produced naturally by simply letting a brine solution dry in the sun. Or it can be produced by heating and vacuum-drying in a factory. Mined salt is simply dug up from the ground.

You can buy Himalayan salt, which is mined; sea salt, which is usually evaporated by the sun; or Morton salt, produced by vacuum evaporation in a factory. Mined and naturally evaporated salts contain trace minerals, which are generally beneficial unless the salt source is contaminated with heavy metals or pollutants—which is unfortunately increasingly a problem. Salts produced by vacuum evaporation are generally devoid of trace minerals, which also means they're less likely to have pollutants. These vacuum-evaporated, more highly processed salts are also much finer and usually have anticaking agents added to prevent them from clumping back

into little salt rocks. The anticaking agents chosen often contain alumi-
num, which is certainly not ideal.

As you can see, there are potential advantages and disadvantages
to each and every kind of salt. In the end, what matters most is you get
enough of it.

RULE #4: DRINK WATER

DO NOT Drink Soda, Juice, Heavily Sweetened Beverages, or Beverages Containing Sucralose or Saccharin

As we know, sugar can cause a lot of health problems. Its insulin-
elevating effect can make you build fat. Its addictive nature can make you
overeat. Sugar's fatburn-blocking effects can cause hypoglycemia that
makes you feel hungry and tired or otherwise bad just a short while after
eating.

Everything that applies to eating sugar applies to drinking it too.
Whether in the form of soda, juice, or heavily sweetened beverages, sugar
has the same effect. Surveys show the average person drinks 200 calories of
juice daily, plus 150 calories of sugary beverages like soda, teas, and coffee.
If your personal sugar intake is anything close to that high, cutting those
350 calories and keeping everything else the same would take off about a
pound every ten days. This one step goes a long way toward improving
your habits.

You might think that drinking reduced-calorie beverages and foods
made with non-sugar sweeteners will help you lose weight. Studies show
that this strategy almost universally fails. The only time low-calorie sweetened products seem to help promote weight loss is when they're part of a
tightly controlled diet program that helps ensure you're not eating more
of something else.

Furthermore, some artificial sweeteners are downright bad for you.
Two stand out in particular as being harmful.

The first, saccharin, is sold under the brand names Sweet 'N Low and
Necta Sweet. This is a carcinogenic molecule that is banned in Canada. I
recommend you avoid saccharin.

The second, sucralose, is sold under the brand names Splenda, ZeroCal, Sukrana, SucraPlus, Cukren, Nevella, and Canderel Yellow. Sucralose is simply sugar that has chlorine molecules added to it, and was shown to cause colon polyps in rats. In spite of the colon problems, the FDA went ahead and approved it. I recommend you avoid sucralose, too.

Newer low-calorie sweeteners that are popping up in beverages are stevia, monk fruit, and coconut sugar. Even though these are natural and won't cause cancer or colon polyps, I recommend you consider limiting or avoiding these as well. The reason in this case has to do with how sweetness itself affects your body and your brain.

We've already discussed how hypoglycemia symptoms are a sign that your brain is addicted to sugar. That's because your brain has been trained to associate sweet taste with energy—and the brain loves getting energy. Your brain is a power-hungry organ. In other words, anything sweet—even if there's no sugar or carbohydrate in it—makes your brain think plenty of energy is on its way. This promotes weight gain in two powerful ways that have nothing to do with calorie intake and everything to do with hormone balance and habit.

First, sweet taste releases fatburn-blocking hormones. It's not just sugar that makes your body release insulin; it's anything with a sweet taste. And remember, insulin slows down the release of fat from your fat closet. In other words, adding an artificial sweetener to water and drinking the sweet-tasting water will block your fatburn even if it has zero calories. Furthermore, whenever you eat or drink something that slows down the release of fat from your fat closet, you can expect to experience hunger in a short while. So drinking artificially sweetened beverages when you're hungry can set you up to be even more hungry a short while later.

Second, in order to repair your metabolic health, you need to retrain your habits. Habits live in your brain. Right now, your brain thinks sweet-tasting foods are the answer to all your brain's energy problems. If you continue to consume sweet-tasting foods or beverages as snacks and when you're hungry, you will not be retraining your brain to look forward to getting energy from fat. And that means you will not be able to change your habits or control your cravings and calorie intake the way you'll need to in order to lose weight and keep it off for good.

So what can you drink instead of these sweet and sugary beverages?

DO Drink Plenty of Water

Crystal clear, clean, refreshing when chilled, and naturally calorie-free, water may be the ultimate weight loss beverage. Our bodies are made of 55 to 60 percent water, and many people don't drink enough.

Though water is clearly essential, there's controversy over how much we actually need. Recommendations range from "just drink when you're thirsty" to eight glasses a day and more if you exercise or spend a lot of time being hot. In my view "just drink when you're thirsty" probably works well when people have perfectly healthy metabolisms and don't take any medication. The rest of us really should pay attention to our water intake and get at least those eight glasses a day, or roughly 80 ounces.

How Drinking Water Helps Weight Loss

Drinking water helps weight loss in several ways.

First and foremost, it's a great way to help curb a snacking habit. If you snack because you're bored, you want a break, or you need to do something with your hands, then a glass of water is a simple snacking-cessation solution.

Furthermore, if you drink two or three cups with meals, the sheer volume helps you to feel full. Let's face it, even though we all know we're supposed to stop eating when we're no longer hungry, some of us don't follow through. It's not that we're gluttons. It's that we don't get the memo. Unlike hunger, which gets our attention the way a dashboard warning light can when it first turns on, the "I'm satisfied" feeling is pretty subtle and easy to miss, more like a dashboard warning light turning off. So we blow right past satisfied and eat until we start to feel pretty darn full—especially at lunch or dinner. Even those of us who have a fully functional appetite regulation center that sends those satiety signals right on time, myself included, may not stop eating until we experience a certain degree of discomfort from being overstuffed. For these folks, two to three full glasses of water with meals becomes an essential part of the solution to curb overeating at meals.

A third way water helps you lose weight is by aiding digestion. A healthy stomach secretes about 2 liters of fluid every day. The pancreas, liver, and small intestine combine to produce another 3½ liters daily. But if your diet has been unhealthy, these organs may not be fully functional. As a result, some people experience problems with recurring nausea alleviated by snacking, which drives you to snack. Others have difficulty digesting certain high-protein or savory foods, which drives them to starches and sweets. For many of these people, the simple recommendation to drink 2 to 3 cups of water with meals has helped reduce their symptoms.

What to Drink If You Can't Drink Just Water

The first priority is to avoid soda, juice, sweet tea, and other high-sugar beverages. The next priority is to avoid anything sweet enough to make you think, *Oh boy, that's sweet.*

What does that leave you with?

For those die-hard, I-can't-drink-water folks among us, I recommend finding products flavored with natural fruit and herb essences. These are zero-calorie beverages with no added sugar and no artificial sweeteners. I've provided a few brand suggestions for these top-of-the-line, high-quality flavored waters, as well as alternatives that are a little sweeter for those folks who need to take baby steps and cut sugar down more gradually.

I recommend finding products flavored with natural fruit and herb essences. Right now the only ones I can find are LaCroix and Hint. No doubt more are on the way.

The following are zero-calorie beverages with no added sugar and no artificial sweeteners.

Best Flavored Sparkling Water
Brand: La Croix, www.lacroixwater.com
Cost: About $20 for twenty-four 12-ounce cans (Amazon, Costco)

Best Flavored Still Water
Brand: Hint
Cost: $17 to $21 per case of twelve 16-ounce bottles.

This brand contains sweeteners, artificial flavors, and glycerin, making it less ideal but still better than soda, juice, and not drinking enough water.

Best Flavor Drops
Brand: SweetLeaf

Flavored stevia drops that you add to sparkling or still water
Cost: About $2.40 for a bottle that makes forty-eight 8-ounce servings.

Do-It-Yourself Flavored Water
Recipe from Deliciously Organic (https://deliciouslyorganic.net
/flavored-water-recipes/)

1 cup fruit, such as citrus or berries
2 sprigs herbs, such as thyme or mint
8 cups water

Combine all ingredients together in a pitcher. Muddle to release the juices
or leave the fruit to float.

Delightful Combinations
Lemon, lime, and orange
Raspberry and lime
Pineapple and mint
Lemon and cucumber
Blackberry and sage
Watermelon and rosemary
Mango and blueberries
Orange and vanilla
Strawberry and basil
Cherry and lime
Blackberry and ginger
Peach and vanilla bean
Honeydew and lime
Pineapple, raspberry, and mint
Peach, lemon, and thyme

Now that you've learned how to make the most of water, let's take a
look at supplements I recommend, which, because of their extreme high
nutrient content, you could consider the opposite of water.

RULE #5: SMART SUPPLEMENTATION

DO Supplement Vitamins and Minerals

Vitamins and minerals are essential nutrients that we need to get from our diet in order to be healthy.

Minerals include calcium, iron, selenium, zinc, iodine, magnesium, copper, phosphorus, and manganese. Sodium and chloride—discussed in Rule #3, "Seek salt"—are also minerals. If you remember your high school chemistry lessons, then some of these minerals will sound familiar. They are all elements listed on the periodic table. All elemental minerals ultimately come from the planet's crust—rocks and stones under the soil. We can mine these elements and we can control what they're associated with, but we cannot create them. Only the universe can.

Vitamins include fat-soluble A, D, E, and K and water-soluble B1, B2, B3, B5, B6, B9, B12, and C. These are organic molecules that are generally made by simple organisms like bacteria and yeasts, or by plants. Plants and microbes in our guts and in the guts of animals we eat are the primary sources of these vitamins.

We're supposed to get all the vitamins and minerals we need by eating a variety of foods, including both plant and animal products. But that's no longer possible for most of us.

Most People Don't Get Enough Vitamins and Minerals

Unfortunately, today the soil is depleted of minerals from generations of conventional farming, which fails to replace what's removed. This is true even for organic food. Organic farming prohibits petrochemical fertilizers and pesticides, but that's no guarantee that the soil is properly fortified with the full spectrum of minerals. Studies have shown that while organically grown food sometimes has more vitamins than conventionally grown, sometimes the opposite is true. It all depends on the farm itself because there is no standard that governs the proper fortification of the soil with minerals.

When plants grow in less-than-ideal soil, they cannot produce the normal amount of vitamins. Compared to vegetables in the 1960s, vegetables today are lower in vitamins of all kinds. What's more, some of the vitamins in raw foods are destroyed by heat. Others are destroyed by UV light. Still others are destroyed during extended storage, and this includes while frozen.

Given the sad state of American food, it shouldn't be surprising that studies show most Americans are falling short of the recommended amounts for multiple vitamins and minerals. Surveys reveal widespread deficiency, which improves as you climb the socioeconomic ladder but fails to reach full sufficiency even in the wealthiest individuals. The human body can deal with a less-than-adequate supply of vitamins and minerals for a little while. But continued deprivation almost always leads to problems.

Our bodies use minerals to build things. Take, for example, bone. Bone is made of calcium and a number of other minerals. When your diet is chronically low in calcium and other minerals required for making bone, your bones can become weak, and will fracture easily. This becomes a problem when someone tries to exercise, or is subjected to trauma.

I had the honor of working with the LA Lakers for several years. One of their young stars suffered a very unusual fracture of his leg due to inadequate mineral intake. Because of the seriousness of the fracture, it was unsure if he would fully recover. Speaking with him, I learned that as a kid he drank milk like crazy, which helped him reach nearly seven feet tall. But in high school he had wrongly been told that dairy was going to make him fat, so he stopped drinking it entirely. His early milk intake helped him build a huge skeleton. And then, when milk was cut out, his diet was unable to properly sustain his massive frame. To help turn around the process of deteriorating bone health, I advised him to get back in the habit of drinking milk. He was very happy to do so and, fortunately for both his health and his career, made a complete and rapid recovery.

REAL MILK: NATURE'S VITAMIN- AND MINERAL-RICH PERFORMANCE BEVERAGE

Not all cow's milk is created equal. I recommend milk from grass-fed cows whenever possible. Called *grass milk*, or *pasture milk*, this variety is hard to find and expensive, but worth every extra penny. You might think all milk comes from cows fed grass, but unfortunately that's not been true for decades. Most cows are fed primarily corn and soy. When cows are fed grass, their milk contains key vitamins you need to build healthy bones, including A and a newly discovered vitamin called K2. Grass milk has more than double the content of brain-building omega-3 fatty acids. When cows are fed corn and soy, their milk has much less of these essential nutrients. Even conventional milk, however, is still a fantastic source of muscle- and bone-building amino acids, minerals, and vitamins.

Vitamins and Minerals Fight Inflammation That Blocks Fatburn

Aside from helping us build healthy tissues, vitamins and minerals also help you regain your ability to burn off body fat.

One of the main uses for minerals in the body is to support antioxidant enzymes. Antioxidant enzymes are critically important for fatburn because they protect your cellular energy-generation centers from inflammation released during the process of burning fat. The more vegetable oil in your body fat, the more inflammation your cells are forced to deal with while burning body fat. All that inflammation eventually makes your cells unnaturally dependent on sugar, as we've already learned. The more antioxidant enzymes you have, the less inflammation your cells will deal with, and the faster you can retrain your cells to burn fat instead of sugar. Everyone who needs to lose weight would benefit from supplementing with the minerals I recommend below to help ensure inflammation-fighting enzymes can handle the stress of burning those stores of toxic vegetable oil.

No matter how well fortified your diet may be with minerals, your body still needs to be able to make repairs whenever and wherever inflammation gets out of control. Vitamins are essential to making those repairs. When inflammation damages important molecules in your cells, like DNA and cell membrane fatty acids, vitamins step in to help. Vitamins C and E work together to fix your cell membranes, while folate, a B vitamin, helps repair DNA. Other vitamins are essential to make other repairs in the cell. Inflammation damages so many cellular structures and disrupts so many metabolic activities that it's important to be sure you have a full range of vitamins in your body at all times to support your metabolic recovery.

It's Best to Get Vitamins and Minerals from Food

Vitamins and minerals consumed in the form of food are more useful to our bodies than those consumed in the form of a pill. For example, studies show that when you try to meet all your calcium requirements from pills rather than food, a good portion of the calcium does not get put to good use. Instead of most of the calcium building bone, as it does when you eat a balanced diet of calcium-rich foods, calcium is redirected to the wrong tissues, like the kidneys, where it can cause kidney stones, or tendons, where it can cause bone spurs. It's like your body can't figure out what to do with calcium unless it comes with the whole package of instructions present in real food.

The same applies to other vitamins and minerals. This is why no expert in their right mind would suggest you'd be fine making a meal of Twinkies and Oreos as long as you swallow handfuls of vitamins and mineral supplements.

The diet that I recommend helps give you a good baseline of nutrition, including most vitamins and minerals. Still, it's hard to get enough. So I recommend taking a small amount of additional vitamins and minerals in the form of a multivitamin and targeted minerals. The small amounts I recommend are going to be beneficial because they are truly supplemental, and not nearly as high as the doses that cause problems.

These are vitamin and mineral supplements I recommend to everyone:

Vitamins

- **Multivitamin.** Mason One a Day is the most balanced multivitamin readily available, containing the closest to 100 percent of most of the vitamins our bodies need. Most other brands are wildly imbalanced with several thousand times the recommended daily allowance (RDA) of some vitamins and a fraction of the RDA of other vitamins.
- **Vitamin D,** which we used to get from sunshine before we built houses and moved indoors. Between 2,000 and 4,000 IU will get your blood level into the normal zone. Example: Carlson Super Daily D3, 2000 IU or 4000 IU. One bottle should last one person one year. This brand uses coconut oil as a vehicle, which is why I recommend it. Most other brands use soy.

Minerals

These are minerals I recommend to everyone to counteract soil depletion:

- **Magnesium oxide,** 250 milligrams. There are many brands available; for example, Nature Made.
- **Zinc picolinate,** 22 milligrams. Example: Solgar.

These are minerals I recommend for special situations:

For Vegans and Folks with Thyroid Disease
- **Iodine:** Especially helpful for anyone with thyroid disease. Maine
  Coast Sea Vegetables Dulse, 2-ounce bag. This particular type of
  seaweed is so high in iodine, it's basically a supplement. Use one
  bag every two months; add to salad, or just chew it when you're
  standing around in the kitchen.

For People Who Do Not Get Three Servings of Dairy on a Daily Basis

A serving of dairy is 8 ounces of milk, 6 ounces of regular yogurt,
4 ounces of cottage cheese, or 1 ounce of hard cheese like cheddar or Swiss.
Three of any combination, plus the calcium from other healthy foods,
should get you to your calcium goal.

Note: Butter, cream, cream cheese, sour cream, half-and-half, and
cheeses made of cream instead of milk, like Brie, are not good sources of
calcium. That's because those are mostly made of the fat, and dairy fat does
not have much calcium. Most of the calcium is bound to casein protein in
the whey component of milk, which makes regular yogurt a better source
of calcium than Greek.

If you cannot get three servings of dairy, I recommend a calcium supplement: calcium citrate, 250 milligrams to 500 milligrams max. You need
about 1000 milligrams daily, but supplementing with more than about 500
milligrams from supplements is associated with kidney stones and bone
spurs, so it's important to make up the rest from dairy and other calcium-
rich foods.

Three Kinds of Supplements That Stand in for Superfoods

In my first book, *Deep Nutrition: Why Your Genes Need Traditional Food*, I identify four categories of foods that all traditional (preindustrial) cultures around the world had in common. They are:

- Fresh food like salads
- Meat on the bone like chicken legs rather than skinless boneless chicken
- Fermented and sprouted foods like live-culture pickles and sprouted grain bread
- Organ meats like liver

These are the original superfoods, and eating them regularly is the best way to optimize your health. As you can see, they're not specific foods but rather entire categories of foods. We all need to eat from all four categories as regularly as possible, but few people actually do. The only one that most people manage to consistently get are the fresh foods. It's not that the other three categories no longer exist; it's that we don't learn how to cook them or how important they are to our growth, health, and well-being.

Fortunately, there are supplements that help fill these nutritional gaps. While ideally you'll eventually be able to get the foods themselves into your body, until then I highly recommend the following three substitutes, discussed below.

Why not supplement all four superfoods? Because there is no substitute for fresh. The supplements that claim to convey the benefits of fresh food are simply not fresh enough to have those benefits. So don't believe the hype and don't waste your hard-earned cash. Take the money you saved from not buying "antioxidant" compounds or supplements based on herbs, like turmeric and garlic, and instead, buy yourself fresh garlic or turmeric, herbs like basil and cilantro, or fix yourself colorful salads.

Cartilage and Collagen Supplements

These supplements help to make up for a diet lacking the nutrients from "meat on the bone." Cartilage and collagen work together to support joint, hair, skin, and nail health, as well as gut health.

While a diet that includes meat on the bone from homemade or store-bought liquid stock is best, the reality is not everyone has time to make bone broth from scratch (or money for the boxed products mentioned next). That's why I highly recommend products such as Kirkland brand organic chicken stock and Pacific Foods organic chicken or beef stock.

As beneficial as these can be, collagen is easily converted to sugar, and so you will experience more benefits from this supplement combination after you have reduced your body's dependence on sugar. I recommend starting these during Phase II of the Fatburn Fix Plan.

Cartilage
FoodScience of Vermont Superior Cartilage
Ancestral Supplements Bovine Tracheal Cartilage

Collagen
CB Supplements Multi Collagen Protein

I suggest you buy both cartilage and collagen supplements as the two of them work best together in more than a 2+2=4 kind of thing—it's more like a 2+2=10 kind of thing.

Probiotic Supplements
These supplements help to make up for a diet lacking the nutrients from fermented and sprouted foods. Prebiotics and probiotics help to support gut and immune system health.

Probiotics are best when consumed in the form of foods like plain whole milk yogurt, lacto-fermented dill pickles or sauerkraut, or kimchi. I recommend plain yogurt because flavored yogurts are loaded with sugar, and when organisms ferment cane sugar, they are less able to support your gut health.

If you don't like any of those foods, you can get probiotics from supplements. When buying supplements, you need to get a good-quality supplement, not the cheap one off the shelf at CVS. The reason for this is they don't stay alive in capsules very long, especially when not refrigerated.

Don't fall for the hype, however. Probiotics are a lucrative industry. There are new brands on the scene every day making all kinds of claims that have little to no factual basis. Additionally, there's no oversight in the supplement industry, so there's no guarantee you're going to get what you are paying for. Fortunately, a few private companies are trying to make up for the lack of oversight. I trust the folks at Consumer Reports to do the best job at keeping up with the changes. Their 2019 report lists the following as their recommended brands.

- BlueBiotics Ultimate Care
- Ultimate Flora Extra Care
- Garden of Life RAW Probiotics
- InnovixLabs Multi-Strain Probiotic
- Vitamin Bounty Pro-25

Organ Meat Supplements

These supplements help to make up for a diet lacking the nutrients from organ meats. Organ meats are truly nutritional powerhouses, concentrated with vitamins, minerals, and other essential nutrients that you don't get in muscle meats. By the way, if you don't eat animal products, herbs and spices are the plant world's near equivalent.

Unfortunately, unless you grew up eating organ meats, you probably won't dive in with enthusiasm. Organ meats are explosively flavorful, and the flavors are so intense they can actually be off-putting. Fortunately, a few highly ethical companies produce very high-quality supplements.

Liver is the most popular of all the organ meats, at least here in the US. Back in the pre–World War II days, before there were any supplements at all, doctors used to recommend liver as a cure for a wide variety of ailments, from anemia to asthma. I myself have seen incredible results in patients who were able to consistently either eat liver or take liver pills.

Liver pills are made of freeze-dried liver. The fancy word for freeze-dried is "desiccated," and that's the best search term to use. The bottles usually recommend you swallow three to six each day. But I recommend one to two per day because that much seems to get the job done.

You'll find lots of brands out there. Try to get something organic and pasture-raised. Two of my favorites are:

- Mother's Best Liver Pills
- Ancestral Supplements

Now that you've learned about the most beneficial supplements, let's take a look at the products that waste your hard-earned cash and can even harm your health.

Do Not Supplement Antioxidants, Phytonutrients, Amino Acids, or Anything Else Not Listed Above

Most supplements I see people spending their money on are a joke. I've seen folks spend hundreds of dollars a month on these products. You'll find that many of the health gurus on the web, including many alternative or naturopathic doctors, are selling supplemental products. You can't get out of a health food store without passing row upon row of these products. Why are they so popular?

Follow the money.

Supplements are an unregulated industry. That means the words on the bottle mean practically nothing. Most testimonials are paid for, and most folks who say how any given supplement has been so amazing for their health are actually the salespeople. Supplements are also easy to make, and easy to ship and store—much easier than real food. One industry insider jokingly told me years ago that everyone who owns a lawn mower has everything they need to start a line of herbal products.

Most of the supplements marketed to bodybuilders, like alanine, creatine, and lecithin—just to name a few—are simply ordinary components of food that have been concentrated into a pill. Your body can make many of them and has little need for the rest. Some are downright dangerous. A few years back mangosteen was marketed as a weight loss aid. One of my patients ended up in the emergency room with an episode of atrial fibrillation that fortunately reversed when she stopped the supplement. The literature is littered with examples of people injured and disfigured from supplements they assumed were safe.

Protein powders are extremely popular. Most are by-products of other industries and also used for animal feed, fertilizer, or industrial manufacturing. Whey protein powder, for instance, is a by-product of making yogurt. It used to be sold to pig farms and institutions for the old and infirm because it was cost-effective. Now it's sold as a health product. Greek yogurt produces more whey, and the rise of Greek yogurt parallels the rise of whey protein powder in stores.

If you want high-protein foods, eat meat, including poultry, fish, and other animal-based products. If you don't eat these foods, your best choices are traditionally produced, plant-based high-protein foods such as fermented (not factory-synthesized) tofu (also called bean curd or soy cheese), tempeh, and seitan. If you want more whey protein, drink more milk. Ricotta cheese is made from whey and tastes great mixed with peanut butter and a little honey, or as the base for a veggie smoothie.

Antioxidant supplements have been hyped for several decades now. The success of this industry rests entirely on consumer ignorance. As I mentioned, the most important antioxidants in your body are the antioxidant enzymes your body makes in abundance as long as your diet contains enough nutrients, especially the minerals previously discussed. The antioxidant compounds you can get from foods serve to protect the food during the cooking process and potentially also during digestion. What's more, most of the antioxidant supplements marketed to prevent aging are too old to actually function, having sat on the shelves for months or more and degraded over time. Another thing these companies don't tell you is that these antioxidants simply do not work in isolation. You need a broad spectrum. And the spectrum is only available to you if you eat a variety of fresh foods. When taken alone, these supplements can actually have the opposite of the intended effect, promoting oxidation and inflammation rather than shutting it down.

I could go on. But others already have; books have been written about the dangers of this Wild West of human experimentation. I would much rather see you take the money you were spending on supplements and spend it on tasty food.

Speaking of tasty food, now that you've mastered the background material you need to follow the plan, let's get you started down that road to lasting health. In Phase I, you'll be doing just that.

12

Phase I

Metabolic Rehab: Baby Steps

IN THIS CHAPTER YOU'LL LEARN TO

- Gain freedom from snacks.
- Take small steps toward long-term habit change.
- Make meals that keep your energy up between meals.

The key to your success is making you feel better, and we'll do that right away by giving you more energy.

In Phase I, Baby Steps, I want you to focus on eliminating all eleven hypoglycemia symptoms that may be making you feel like you need to boost your energy with a snack. We'll accomplish this by teaching you to make meals that provide you with lasting energy, thus giving you more energy between meals so that you don't feel the need to snack.

HOW TO MAKE ENERGIZING MEALS

If you're accustomed to fruits, juices, sweet-tasting beverages, donuts, cereal, muffins, bagels, pasta, rice, or any sweet or starchy substances with any of your meals, you now know that those foods can make you tired and prone to overeating. Now it's time to begin training yourself how to live without them. The key will be learning to swap out energy-draining ingredients for energizing clean-burning fats and slow-digesting carbs.

This chapter will give you guidance on making all your meals with clean-burning fats and slow-digesting carbs. The idea is that you'll be able to make breakfast and lunch in minutes and spend just a little more time on dinner. We're going to do both by teaching you about the healthiest ingredients that only need a little bit of help to be transformed into a meal. You'll also learn to use the upgraded versions of a number of convenient, processed foods. These upgraded items are made by more conscientious companies whose products are superior for one of three reasons: (1) they don't use toxic fats, (2) they use sprouted grains and seeds instead of highly refined, nonnutritive flours, and (3) they don't use massive amounts of sugar.

However, I do not expect you to rush to the store and buy everything I recommend in this chapter or make changes to all three meals right now. Some people can. Some people prefer to start out running and dive right in headfirst. Very often these go-getter folks are foodies or already have broad kitchen skills or at least have ample time for learning. The vast majority of us need to take it slowly. For people who are not very comfortable in the kitchen, or who have family members who need special meals, or who have sensitive digestive systems, I strongly recommend you adapt just a few of the recommendations at a time.

Right now you probably have a kitchen full of familiar but unhealthy foods and a body full of metabolic disruption. We need to teach you to shop for new foods, to prepare food differently, and if you snack, we also need you to change your eating habits.

It's perfectly OK to start with just one change, something as simple as using real cream in your coffee instead of sweetened creamers. Or making your lunches with nitrate-free deli meat. Or buying olive oil to make your own salad dressing. I would also ask you to commit to making one new change with every shopping trip as you go forward, buying at least one new kind of upgraded food each time you buy groceries, gradually weaning off the processed foods made with vegetable oils and too much starchy carb and sugar.

PHASE I: BABY STEPS GOALS

Phase I is all about preparing your metabolism for Phase II so you can lose weight permanently. The first step toward that goal is snacking cessation. To get a handle on the issue, you need to consciously take notice of how much grazing and off-the-cuff eating you've been doing. Instead of snacking, I want you to concentrate on eating meals instead.

I want you to concentrate on building the kinds of meals that will sustain your energy between meals. So in this chapter we're going to help sustain your energy by teaching you two swap-outs. First, you'll eat slow-digesting carbs instead of starchy carbs and sweets. And second, you'll eat plenty of healthy, clean-burning fats instead of energy-sapping vegetable oils.

To avoid the starchy carbs and sweets you will be limiting and ideally avoiding anything made with flour and anything really sweet, including most large pieces of fruit and cookies, cakes, pastries, donuts, muffins, etc. Giving up these foods will be difficult—I'm not gonna lie—but it's partly because they've become your habit. If you commit to forming a new habit in place of the old habit, you can pull it off. And don't worry about hunger because including slow-digesting carbs and clean-burning fats will make your meals more sustaining. The healthy fats you will be enjoying will be slowly released from your digestive system and provide you with energy for hours. The slow-digesting carbs provide a little bit of the sugar-based energy that some people with very damaged metabolisms still need. The energy from these foods will sustain you so that you do not feel hypoglycemia, which is essential to accomplishing the Phase I goal of complete snacking cessation.

Popular clean-burning fats to consider buying next time you shop:

- Avocados
- Avocado oil mayonnaise
- Coconut cream
- Dairy fats: butter, cream or half-and-half, cream cheese (full-fat), sour cream (full-fat)
- Nut butters: almond, peanut

Popular slow-digesting carbs to consider buying next time you shop:

- Sprouted grain bread (usually sold in the freezer section, keep chilled)
- Yellow corn tortillas (made with corn masa, not flour, and these are generally fat-free, so no bad oils)
- Nuts: almond, cashew, pistachio, pecan (avoid any vegetable oils)
- Seeds: chia, hemp, pumpkin, sunflower (avoid any vegetable oils)
- Salad condiments: sun-dried tomatoes, olives, capers, artichoke hearts, roasted or pickled beets, palm hearts (avoid any vegetable oils)

Here's what I mean by simple swap-outs. You can get clean-burning fat by using butter on your toast instead of jelly. Or by buying natural peanut butter made with just peanuts and salt, instead of peanut butter made with sugar and hydrogenated oil. You can make burgers without the bun, and if you can't find ground beef that's not super lean, make it a cheeseburger to get your clean-burning fats. Buy avocado oil mayo so you can enjoy sandwiches on sprouted grain bread, including egg and tuna salads. Make more vegetables at dinner and less rice, pasta, bread, or potato so that you don't even miss those insulin-spiking starches.

WHAT'S INCLUDED?

I'm not going to fill this chapter with a lot of detailed recipes for dishes you may or may not even end up liking. Instead, I'm going to give you easy-to-read tables of ideas on how to make mealtime upgrades by swapping out ingredients or assembling foods into extremely easy dishes. I'll also give you more detailed instructions for just a few essential recipes.

#GOALS: TRICKS TO MAKE HABIT CHANGE EASIER

For the most part I don't like to ask people to use willpower to sustain a healthy way of eating. We only have so much willpower, and I don't want you to use it all up. So in general, this program leverages a little bit of willpower to create a lot of beneficial changes. Snacking is one of those habits where we will need to use a little bit of willpower to change the habit, and it will definitely leverage a lot of beneficial change.

Changing habits is actually easier if you don't think about it as giving up something, but rather as changing one behavior to another. It's easier if you think about swapping a snacking habit for a different habit.

One of the main reasons smokers gain weight when they quit is they often replace a habit that takes them outside to socialize with other smokers with a habit that usually involves eating. I'm not suggesting you start smoking, but that you come up with a new habit that can help you achieve another healthy goal you might have, like being more active, more organized, or spending more time with friends. For example, let's say your current workplace break habit is to head to the cafeteria. Instead, think about heading somewhere else. Can you walk up a few flights of stairs? Can you find a buddy to talk with or go for a walk with? Maybe you can find a place to stand up while you write out a food shopping list.

You may think it sounds silly for me to suggest your special morning treat can be eliminated by starting some kind of productive activity, and that's fair. But I'm guessing it would sound even sillier to you if I suggested you have to keep snacking forever and ever because once you develop a habit there's no way you'll ever change.

WHAT IS A SNACK, ANYWAY?

Since one of the most important baby steps to take is to cut down and eliminate snacking, let's make sure we define what exactly snacking is. Consuming anything with calories outside of a predefined, planned meal—be it breakfast, lunch, or dinner—counts as a snack. Even if it has zero calories, if it tastes sweet, it counts as a snack. Dessert is a planned post-meal treat, and eating it right after the meal means it's not going to have the fatburn-blocking effects of a snack.

SNACK ATTACK SAFETY

I want you to be confident you can tell the difference between a simple snack attack and a snack attack complicated by hypoglycemia symptoms. A simple snack attack is not associated with any of the eleven hypoglycemia symptoms, and while you may feel a little hungry, it will go away without eating. A complex snack attack will make you feel bad in one of those eleven ways, and it won't quit until you do something to boost your cellular energy. Now might be a good time for you to review the hypoglycemia symptoms in Chapter 9 (Fatburn Assessment Tools).

Each time you feel like you want to snack, I want you to please do a quick mental rundown of those eleven symptoms to determine if you are experiencing a simple snack attack or a snack attack with hypoglycemia complications. This will help you decide if you can safely wait for the snack attack to go away or if you need to treat it.

Later in this chapter I will give you specific ideas of what to eat for breakfast and lunch to prevent those hypoglycemia symptoms.

Beware of zero-calorie claims as well. Even when your snack or beverage has zero calories, if it tastes sweet, it can still make you build fat. This is because the flavors of food impact our hormones, and it's our hormones that change when we train our metabolism to build fat by snacking— just as bodybuilders train their metabolism to build lean tissue by working out.

But I LOVE Snacking! You Seriously Need Me to Stop ALL Snacks?!?

If your day is made significantly brighter by snacks, then it's not practical to try to stop all snacks on day one. Let's start you out with a smaller goal.

ACTION STEPS TO SNACKING FREEDOM

It's important to note that while zero snacking and water-only beverages represent your ultimate goal for Phase I, it may take a few baby steps to get to that goal. Let me give you two examples of common challenges and action steps to take.

Give Up Soda

In Chapter 11, discussing the "Drink water" rule, I provided links to a few options for those of you who are ready to give up your soda but not ready to drink only water. This is a good baby step since, even though they block fatburn, the weight-building effect of no-and low-calorie sweet-tasting beverages is less than for caloric beverages. The beverages I recommend in Chapter 11 are not heavily sweetened and block fatburn less powerfully than those that taste sweeter.

Eat Snacks With a Meal

Another baby step may simply be putting off any snacking you do in the morning until the afternoon. As you learned in Chapter 6, the morning cortisol pulse makes it crucial to avoid snacking in the morning. So for example, say you normally bring a snack to work and haven't paid much attention to when you snack, start planning on holding off on that snack until afternoon. (If you can hold off all day, even better.)

Drink Coffee With a Meal

Many of my patients eat a fairly light breakfast or snack before they leave in the morning and then drink a sweet or caloric coffee (with sugar or cream or coffee creamer, for example) an hour or so later. An action step to take here is to consolidate those calories by consuming your breakfast and coffee *together* in one sitting. Or you can drink the coffee at lunch. Whenever you can turn two episodes of calorie consumption into one, you're improving your metabolic health.

Depending on how hungry you are in the morning, you could consider drinking the coffee in the morning and consuming nothing else. In this case you will be holding off on the snack until lunchtime and eating it as part of your lunch.

Graze on Clean-Burning Fats

If you're not in the habit of eating three meals a day because you graze on the run, then a good baby step for you may simply be to eat more healthy fats with your first "graze."

So for example, instead of having a low-fat yogurt or a banana on the run, have a slice of cheese or a small handful of macadamia nuts. The healthy fats will provide your cells with a clean-burning fuel to energize your daily activity. Because your cells get so much energy from the healthy fats, you may find it easier to make it all the way to lunch without grazing on anything else.

Drink Black Coffee or Tea Instead of Eating a Snack

Black coffee and tea are essentially noncaloric. So if you have a habit of snacking at a certain time, drinking a caffeinated, unsweetened beverage like black coffee or unsweetened tea instead can help you get past the craving in a healthy way. Any beverage with zero calories and little to no sweetness can serve the same function, including the unsweetened, naturally flavored waters like those you learned about in the discussion of Rule #4, "Drink water."

BUILDING YOUR MEALS

The two most important considerations in Phase I are to be sure you are getting clean-burning fats and slow-digesting carbs with every meal. Great sources of clean-burning fats you can add to familiar foods are nut butters, avocado, coconut flakes or coconut cream, macadamia nuts, dairy butter, cream (or half-and-half), cream cheese, eggs, and breakfast sausage or bacon. Great sources of clean-burning carb you use to build familiar meals are sprouted grain toast or English muffins, nut butters, starchy nuts like cashews and pecans, chia seeds and hemp seeds, soft corn tortilla shells (made with corn masa, not corn flour), and beans.

RESETTING YOUR STOMACH CLOCK

After following the plan for a few weeks, you should be able to go all morning and all afternoon without snacking and not feel hungry. If that hasn't happened for you, if you find yourself giving in to snack attacks, it may be time to consider your stomach clock.

As you know, your stomach has an alarm clock. If you've had a habit of snacking, you've set your alarm to go off around the time you usually snack. If your alarm clock rings quietly, you may not hear it on a busy day. But if it's a slow day, you'll feel compelled to eat something.

No matter your actual age, your stomach has the mind of an infant. It wants what it wants, and it wants it now. What I'm saying is that if you have trained your stomach that when it asks for food it gets food, then you may need to have a conversation with your stomach the next time the alarm goes off. Be firm and gentle, but you need to be consistent—just like with a baby when you're trying to wean it off nighttime feedings, for example. Just ignore it, drink a big glass of water, get busy doing something productive, and it will stop bugging you. If you ignore it for a few days and then give in, you've just reversed all that training you accomplished.

And it's very important to remember that it's only safe to ignore hunger when it is not associated with any of the eleven hypoglycemia symptoms.

EXTRACT YOUR SWEET TOOTH

Another goal of this phase is to start to resolve any sugar-addiction issues that you may have.

Most people know if they have a sweet tooth, although it's common to be in denial about whether or not their sweet tooth is under control. I used to drink an equivalent of a quarter cup of sugar in my fancy coffee shop coffee every day, and that coffee confection was the only meal I looked forward to. No matter how much my husband was slaving over dinner, it never occupied my mind the way a mocha-sugar-blast-o-Frappuccino would. Even still, I never thought my sugar habit was affecting my appetites or cravings, much less my health. In my first season with the LA Lakers working with Dwight Howard, famous for his candy habit at the time, in one of our early conversations he insisted, "I don't eat that much candy." If that was true, it was only relative to what he had in his house— once Howard understood how many ways his candy habit was impairing his performance and agreed to an intervention, his assistants carted out boxes and boxes of candy.

You will be ready to cut back on your sugar before you know it. In fact, for me the hardest thing about cutting back was simply deciding I would do it. The key to your success will not be going cold turkey. While going cold turkey works for some when quitting cigarettes and alcohol, it rarely works with sugar.

Your path to freedom from sugar addiction looks like this:

Step 1. Consolidate your sweet consumption to one treat per day only. If you keep candy stashed in your purse, your car, your living room, and nosh on a little something sweet all throughout the day, there's no way you're going to sustain a no-sugar policy. You have to make a pact with yourself to demolish your stash houses. Some tricks that can help are chewing sugarless gum and sipping on some unsweetened flavored water or unsweetened herbal tea. You can have one sweet treat per day, ideally at dinner (as dessert), so make it something you really like.

Step 2. Now reduce the sweetness in that treat. If you normally eat milk chocolate, make it dark chocolate. If you normally have cookies and ice cream, cut the amount in half or find a brand that has half the total carbohydrates and sugars. If you normally have soda, try a flavored kombucha. If you normally have a sweet cocktail, make it less sweet—or drink a slightly sweet dessert wine. If you are someone who loves baking and you make your desserts yourself, you can cut the sugar in the recipe you use. This process will take some careful consideration in order to find something that works for you and, yes, some willpower in order to stick to.

Step 3. If you've been in the habit of eating sweets all day, you will feel better including a small portion of slow-digesting carb at meals a few days a week along with the clean-burning fats.

I don't recommend switching to artificial sweeteners for this purpose; aside from sustaining the sweet-taste addiction, the fact is you don't get any calories for free. When it comes to dessert treats, most artificially sweetened foods have just as many total calories because although you're eating less sugar, you're eating relatively more of the other ingredients.

Some people who have been sugar addicts can limit themselves to less than 100 calories per day of sweet treats if and only if these treats are portioned strictly so that you open only one container, for example, or break off one square of chocolate. And if you find yourself slipping back, finishing off two or three squares on a regular basis, then it's time to cut out sweets entirely again for a little while.

PHASE I BREAKFAST IDEAS

The best breakfast meals are high in fat, not dominated by sweet taste, and low in both carb and protein. My breakfast for the past twenty years has been a cup of milk, a lot of cream, and cold-brewed coffee. In other words, the vast majority of calories are coming from fat. An egg or breakfast sausage or bacon are examples of the highest-protein foods I'd recommend for breakfast. On the topic of eggs, any egg dish is going to be healthy, so if you have time to cook, at least peel a hard-boiled egg and take advantage of that. This chapter will focus more on breakfast ideas that you don't need to cook, and we'll dive more into eggs and breakfast meats in the next chapter.

In Phase I, you will ideally be avoiding juices and all fruits other than berries (like blueberries and raspberries) and limiting those to an eighth of a cup or less at breakfast and a quarter cup or less all day. It's best to avoid protein powders at breakfast time as well, since an unhealthy metabolism will end up converting much of the energy in those highly processed, rapidly absorbed proteins to either sugar or fat. If you feel better having a little protein at breakfast, use a protein-rich whole food like eggs, cheese, tofu, and breakfast meats.

Let's start out with a table of common breakfast items and their upgraded solutions. This list includes some of the most common breakfast items with possible replacements. It's not meant to be an exhaustive list, merely examples of easy and familiar swap-outs.

Popular breakfast options that provide plenty of healthy fat and not too much carb or protein:

PHASE I SAMPLE BREAKFAST OPTIONS

INSTEAD OF THIS	TRY THIS
Oatmeal	SLOW CARB CHIA BOWL
Cereal	SLOW CARB YOGURT PARFAIT
Protein or Energy Bar	UPGRADED BARS
Smoothie	HIGH ENERGY BREAKFAST SMOOTHIE
Toast, Pancakes, or Waffles	SPROUTED GRAIN TOAST
foo foo Coffee	COFFEE WITH CREAM AND STEVIA
Juice	WHOLE MILK or UNSWEETENED ALMOND MILK
Fruit	HERBAL TEA

BREAKFAST OPTION DETAILS

Instead of Oatmeal . . .

Oatmeal has too much carb and not enough healthy fat to sustain your energy.

. . . Try a Slow Carb Chia Bowl

Slow Carb Chia Bowls contain slow-digesting carbohydrate, and you will add good fats. Per serving, start with 2 tablespoons chia and ½ to ¾ cup almond, coconut, or cow's milk. The precise ratio will depend on the variety of chia seed you buy, so start out with ½ cup and add more if the texture is not to your liking. Stir together, allow to sit for a few minutes to let the seeds start to expand into gel, then stir again to separate the seeds completely and prevent clumping. If chia texture bothers you, a Vitamix blender will make it smooth, like pudding. Chill in fridge covered for two to twenty-four hours. Before serving or bringing to work, top with 1 tablespoon hemp seed and your favorite toppings (for ideas see Topping Combos for Phase I Breakfast and Lunch on page 244).

Instead of Cereal . . .

Most cereals have too much carb and often bad oils as well, even granola.

. . . Try a Slow Carb Yogurt Parfait

This Slow Carb Yogurt Parfait has plenty of healthy fats from the cream, a little bit of both protein and slow-digesting carb from the yogurt and nuts. Use 6 to 8 ounces of plain whole milk or regular or Greek yogurt with optional ⅛ cup whipped cream or 1½ teaspoons sour cream and your favorite toppings (for ideas see Topping Combos for Phase I Breakfast and Lunch on page 244). If you like cottage cheese, try the same toppings on 4 to 6 ounces of cottage cheese.

Instead of Protein Bars and Energy Bars . . .

Granola bars, fiber bars, breakfast bars, and protein and energy bars generally have bad oils and too much carb. There are a few upgraded options that are the exception to the rule, and more brands appearing on the market daily.

. . . Try Upgraded Bars

The best bars are going to have good fats and less than 10 grams of net carbohydrate.

Best brands: Primal Kitchens, Keto Bars

Widely available brands: Kind bars

Instead of a Smoothie . . .

Most smoothies, even green smoothies, have too much fruit to be a healthy breakfast option and not enough fat to sustain you between meals.

. . . Try a High-Energy Breakfast Smoothie

This High-Energy Breakfast Smoothie contains plenty of healthy fat and just a little protein and carb. Per serving, start with 1 cup of whole milk or unsweetened almond milk, and add 2 to 3 tablespoons of dairy cream or coconut cream, and 6 to 10 ice cubes. Alternatively, use half an avocado and ¾ cup full-fat canned coconut milk.

Flavor with 1 tablespoon cocoa powder and an optional small amount of fruit such as half a banana OR ¼ cup frozen strawberries (though stevia would be preferable); vanilla or almond extract; and a dash of spice like nutmeg or cinnamon.

Instead of Toast, Pancakes, and Waffles . . .

Most toast, pancakes, and waffles contain too much carbohydrate, and the syrup or jelly adds even more.

. . . Try Sprouted Grain Toast

Sprouted grain toast has slow-digesting carbohydrate, and the spread offers plenty of healthy fat plus a little protein. Toasted Ezekiel or other sprouted grain bread 'n' spread.

Avocado Toast

Slice half an avocado, distribute over toast. Optionally, drizzle with coconut cream and a dash of salt.

Butter Blend Toast

1 tablespoon grass-fed butter, plus 1 tablespoon almond butter, on 1 slice sesame (or any flavor) Ezekiel sprouted grain bread (Ezekiel bread is sold in the freezer section of the store), toasted

2 tablespoons peanut butter/coconut oil blended together on half an Ezekiel cinnamon raisin English muffin, toasted

Goat Cheese and Sun-Dried Tomato Toast

Sprouted grain bread, toasted, with 1½ ounces feta cheese stirred or blended together with 1½ ounces cream cheese, topped with 1 to 2 tablespoons sun-dried tomatoes snipped into pieces with cooking shears or chopped fine

Salmon Delight

2 tablespoons grass-fed cream cheese and 1 ounce smoked salmon on 1 slice seven-grain Ezekiel sprouted grain bread or dark Bavarian rye bread, toasted

Variations: Add fresh tomato slices and/or capers in addition to or instead of salmon.

Instead of foo foo Coffee . . .

Coffee actually helps you burn fat, so no need to cut that out. So-called creamers often contain bad fats, and flavored creamers are usually high in sugar. Flavored coffee confections sold at chains such as Dunkin' Donuts and Starbucks are loaded with sugar and, usually, unhealthy fats.

. . . Try Coffee with Cream and Stevia

For each cup of coffee, add ⅛ to ¼ cup cow's milk cream or half-and-half, ideally from pasture-fed cows (Organic Valley is a national brand, but there are many more available locally in health food stores). Flavored coffee beans go a long way to enhance the flavor experience. A stevia brand with no unpleasant aftertaste is SweetLeaf.

Instead of Juice . . .

Most juices are very high in sugar. A glass of all-natural OJ, for example, has as much sugar as a can of soda.

. . . Try Whole Milk or Unsweetened Almond Milk

The best milk comes from pastured cows. Organic Valley sells their Grassmilk nationwide. Unsweetened almond milk is another great option if you don't like dairy. Works great to wash down an upgraded breakfast bar.

Instead of Fruit . . .

An apple or banana has more sugar than a Hershey's bar. Most fruits are too big and too loaded with sugar to eat more than a quarter cup or so at breakfast. Berries and melons are your best option, and if you can, try to hold off till lunch or dessert because, as we learned, sugar does the most damage to your fatburn in the morning.

. . . Try Herbal Tea

If you need a little fruity taste in the morning, herbal tea bags that you brew yourself contain zero calories and no sugar and you can find them in fruity flavors. If you need a little sweetness, add a drop of liquid stevia.

PHASE I LUNCH IDEAS

These lunch ideas are all similar to breakfast in concept: no toxic oils, plenty of healthy fat, a little slow-digesting carb and whole-food protein.

Something else to consider at lunch is getting salt, which is important, as we learned in Rule #3 in the last chapter. Many people notice that getting plenty of salt at lunch in combination with slow carbs and/or clean-burning fats helps keep their energy up all afternoon. Another factor that will help your alertness in the afternoon has to do with the size of the meal. When we eat a lot of food, we tend to get sleepier than when we eat less, so it's important to not overdo your lunch.

If you've developed a habit of ordering a salad for lunch, that's great! Just bring your own olive, roasted peanut, or sesame oil and vinegar to work, and add ⅛ teaspoon of salt. Be sure to ask the folks supplying your salad to hold their dressing (unless you know it's made with a healthy oil and not any of the vegetable oils).

Popular lunch options that provide plenty of healthy fat and not too much carb or protein:

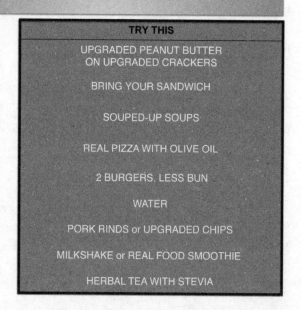

PHASE I SAMPLE LUNCH OPTIONS

INSTEAD OF THIS	TRY THIS
Vending Machine Snacks	UPGRADED PEANUT BUTTER ON UPGRADED CRACKERS
Take-Out Sandwich	BRING YOUR SANDWICH
Noodle Soup	SOUPED-UP SOUPS
Cheap Pizza	REAL PIZZA WITH OLIVE OIL
Burger & Fries	2 BURGERS, LESS BUN
Soda	WATER
Regular Chips	PORK RINDS or UPGRADED CHIPS
Protein Smoothie	MILKSHAKE or REAL FOOD SMOOTHIE
Fruit	HERBAL TEA WITH STEVIA

LUNCH OPTION DETAILS

Instead of Vending Machine Snacks . . .

Unless you work for a company like the one I work for, with a CEO who truly values your health, chances are your vending machines are full of candy bars and junk. Even the peanut butter crackers contain toxic fats and too much carb.

Protein bars also aren't ideal; most protein bars are made from dehydrated and oxidized proteins that your body does not deal with very well, which leads to skin and joint problems. If you are diabetic, your liver will rapidly convert these powders into glucose through the process of gluconeogenesis, so they will elevate your blood sugar.

. . . Try Upgraded Peanut Butter on Upgraded Crackers

The same bars I recommended for breakfast would be suitable for lunch, as would peanut butter crackers you make yourself. Many stores offer fresh ground peanut butter with roasted peanuts and salt as the sole ingredients.

Smucker's makes an organic, all-natural peanut butter, available under $4 at most grocery stores (and online retailers).

Almond butter rarely contains anything but almonds and salt. Mara-Natha organic almond butters come in raw, roasted, crunchy, and creamy.

These crackers are selected because they contain no inflammation-promoting, toxic fats.

- Mary's Gone Crackers, original. Very flavorful, due to many toasted seeds.
- Ak-Mak crackers. Very simple: wheat flour, sesame oil, salt. Thick and sturdy, good for spreading stuff onto. They call themselves a "cracker bread."
- Carr's brand crackers. Caution: Just three of their flavors are free of the toxic fats: (1) Carr's Table Water Crackers, Original, (2) Carr's Table Water Crackers, Toasted Sesame, and (3) Carr's Whole Wheat Crackers.

Instead of a Take-Out Sandwich . . .

Panera, Subway, Quiznos, and most other fast-food joints all use toxic fat and load up their food with too much refined-flour breads. Arby's is a notable exception that I can actually recommend, because their meats contain no weird fillers and their low-carb options contain zero bread. Still, it's almost always best to bring your own.

. . . Try Bringing Your Sandwich

Whether or not your mom packed you lunch for school, now that you're a grownup, you can consider if you'd like to get in the habit of packing one yourself. As you make your transition, you can use two slices of bread if that makes life easier. But as you move through Phase I, you may find you only need one.

Almond Apple Ham and Cheddar

1 tablespoon almond butter, 1½ ounces deli-sliced cheddar, 1½ ounces deli ham, 2 leaves romaine lettuce, about 3 thin apple slices (enough to cover the sandwich), 2 slices sprouted grain bread (toasted to reduce crumbling)

500 Calories; Carb, 33g (Fiber, 8g); Protein, 21g; Fat, 26g

Parisian Antipasto Sandwich

1 slice sprouted grain bread, 1 to 2 ounces thinly sliced Brie cheese, 2 ounces chicken-breast cold cuts (thinner slices are often tastiest), ½ ounce prosciutto, 2 to 3 sun-dried tomatoes snipped fine with cooking shears or chopped or roasted red peppers sliced long and thin

280 Calories; Carb, 15g (Fiber, 3g); Protein, 21g; Fat, 13g

Bavarian Subway Sandwich, California Style and Chips

1 slice Bavarian rye bread, 1½ ounces chicken deli slices or rotisserie chicken, 2 slices salami, a quarter of an avocado, 2 tablespoons sliced pepperoncini (Mezzetta), 1 slice provolone cheese

Melt together in the microwave for 30 seconds. Then add 1 tablespoon mayo. Chips: ½ ounce pork rinds.

460 Calories; Carb, 24g (Fiber, 4 g); Protein, 24 g; Fat, 29g. Sprouted grain version has Carb, 20g (Fiber, 5g).

Open-Face Reuben on Rye

Place 2 ounces of Swiss cheese evenly onto toasted dark Bavarian rye. Heat in microwave or toaster oven till cheese starts to melt, then add 2 ounces corned beef (also works great with ham and turkey). Meanwhile, stir together ½ tablespoon each sweet relish and mayo with 1 teaspoon ketchup (or mustard for turkey) and ¼ teaspoon horseradish. Optionally top with 2 ounces well-drained sauerkraut and heat for a short while longer to blend flavors.

510 Calories; Carb, 19g (Fiber, 1g); Protein, 26g; Fat, 36g

Superfoods Gone Crackers!

One of the healthiest ready-to-eat foods in the entire universe of foods is liver pâté, or any kind of semi-spreadable meat product that includes liver, especially when from pastured animals. 3 ounces liverwurst, head-cheese, or braunschweiger (see "Shopping List for Phase I" on page 251). Spread carefully or simply place to avoid cracking on Carr's Original Water Crackers. Dollop each cracker with a quick dressing from 2 tablespoons avocado oil mayo, 2 tablespoons mustard, and ¼ teaspoon horseradish.

480 Calories; Carb, 18g (Fiber, 3g); Protein, 15g; Fat, 40g

Instead of Noodle Soup . . .

Ramen and instant noodle soup are perfect examples of what's wrong with food, loaded with vegetable oils, fake flavoring agents, and flours. Even if you're nuts for noodles now, your energy will be much better when you make the swap-out below.

. . . Try Souped-Up Soups

A few companies make some of their soups without toxic oils. Hallelujah. But no one company makes all of their soups with healthy oils, so you still need to read the ingredients to avoid them. The soups are low-fat, so that just one serving will leave you hungry, while more than one serving contains too much sugar. So the best solution is adding something more substantial to a single serving to soup them up.

Roasted Red Pepper and Sausage Lentil Soup (single serving, 5 minutes)

Pacific Foods makes a Vegetable Lentil and Roasted Red Pepper Soup that goes great with a ready-to-eat sausage like nitrate-free options from Publix GreenWise or Applegate Farms. Just slice the sausage and heat together with the soup on a stovetop or in a microwave.

Kale and Millet Sausage Soup (single serving, 5 minutes)

Pacific Foods also makes a White Bean Kale & Millet Soup that goes well with ready-to-eat nitrate-free grass-fed beef hot dogs, nitrate-free Italian sausage, provolone cheese, or mozzarella. Just slice the sausage and heat together with the soup on a stovetop or in the microwave.

Instead of Cheap Pizza . . .

Most pizza joints and chains use "olive oil blends," meaning there's a tiny amount of olive oil mixed in with the vegetable oil. If you can find one that uses pure olive oil in their sauces, order theirs. Otherwise take a few shortcuts and make your own.

. . . Try Real Pizza with Olive Oil

Shortcut #1: buy ready-made dough. Shortcut #2: buy already shredded or sliced cheese, pepperoni, and stir-fry veggies. Now you just need the sauce. Use Ragú's Simply line or make your own. Makes a great dinner when you load it up with precooked ground beef or sausage.

Instead of Soda . . .

There's nothing good about soda.

. . . Try Water

There's nothing bad about water. If you don't like the lack of taste, see Chapter 11 (Five Rules That Fix Your Fatburn) on how to add flavor to your water.

Instead of Regular Chips, Popcorn, and Other Snacks . . .

Most regular chips are loaded with toxic oils. This even includes "healthy" chips like Sun Chips, veggie chips, and baked chips.

. . . Try Upgraded Chips and Pork Rinds

A few companies are making chips and popcorn in olive oil, avocado oil, coconut oil, and even ghee. You can buy these online and have them shipped if your local stores don't carry them yet. Chips are high in carb even when fried in healthy oil, so it's easy to overeat them. Because of this, I don't recommend keeping even upgraded chips around unless you can limit your intake to 1 ounce per day. The trick to finding them is googling in quotes "ghee popcorn" or "olive oil chips."

Pork rinds are a classic low-carb snack. Pork rinds are simply pig skin fried in pig fat to crispness. They contain 0 carb and plenty of protein.

Instead of a Protein Smoothie . . .

Most protein smoothies are made with powders. Protein powders get absorbed fast enough to spike insulin, and when your metabolism is not healthy, it will convert most of the protein into sugar or body fat.

Protein powders are processed-food versions of proteins that are definitely a step down in terms of nutritional value relative to the value they would bring to your body when consumed directly from their original source. Whey protein powder is abundant and cheap because it's a byproduct of cheese and yogurt making. These powders can block fatburn because they spike insulin, very much like bread made from refined wheat flour spikes insulin more than sprouted grain bread made from the intact wheat berry.

. . . Try a Milk Shake or Real-Food Smoothie . . .

With your own blender, you can leave out the powder and blend in real food instead. Start with any kind of milk and blend in the real-food protein sources below.

Top Four Real-Food Protein Sources for Shakes

If you're a protein shake aficionado, try experimenting with these four options instead of the powder.

Tofu is the blandest—it goes with nearly everything. Silken tofu is the softest and blandest but is lower in protein than firmer tofus.

Ricotta cheese is the next blandest, and its creamy richness makes it my top choice.

Greek yogurt is nearly as bland as ricotta.

Regular plain yogurt has a sourness that works well as a tangy backdrop for a sweet-and-sour experience.

Here's a couple easy recipes to make you a real-food milk shake or smoothie convert:

Raspberries 'n' Cream

I cup full-fat ricotta
½ cup frozen raspberries (make sure to use unsweetened)
Dash vanilla extract
Dash salt
2–3 drops liquid stevia if desired
(Cal 490, Protein 29 gm, Carb 22 gm, Fiber 8 gm)

Chocolate Peanut Butter Bliss

4 ounces firm tofu, raw
2 tablespoons natural peanut butter, salted
2 tablespoons cocoa powder, unsweetened
½ cup whole milk (or almond milk)
420 Calories; Protein, 29 g; Carb, 29 g (Fiber, 12 g)

Low-Carb Smoothie Bowl

For the base, use ½ cup of soft tofu or ½ to I cup of plain Greek yogurt instead of protein powder. The yogurt is sour, so it works well if you're in the mood for a sweet-and-sour experience, whereas the tofu is totally bland. Sweeten with ¼ cup frozen strawberries or blueberries and stevia. Flavor with vanilla extract and nutmeg, or with cinnamon and anise (a.k.a. fennel seeds).

Alternatively, instead of yogurt or tofu for the base, blend ½ cup frozen cauliflower rice with I medium avocado and 2 to 3 tablespoons full-fat canned coconut milk or milk (almond or cow's), plus more as needed.

Instead of Fruit . . .

As with breakfast, fruit is just too full of sugar to be a healthy addition to lunch. But if you just need a little something sweet, try herbal tea with stevia.

. . . Try Herbal Tea with Stevia

Works great for lunch as well as breakfast. Tastes best chilled over ice.

MY FAVORITE DAIRY PARFAIT

These are a few of my all-time favorite ways to jazz up yogurt to make breakfast, lunch, or even a super healthy after-dinner treat.

Greek Yogurt with Chocolate, Coconut, and Curried Cashews

6 ounces nonfat Greek yogurt (you can use full-fat if you like it and can find it, but this version gets you plenty of fat thanks to the toppings, so nonfat is fine) with 2 tablespoons curry-coconut-spiced cashews, 2 tablespoons coconut flakes, and 1 tablespoon cacao nibs. Keep dry ingredients in separate container. You can buy a variety of delicious spiced nuts online from LivingIntentions.com or make your own! If you can't find curry-coconut-spiced cashews, add a sprinkle of Thai curry powder along with regular raw or dry-roasted and salted cashews.

400 Calories; Carb, 22 g (Fiber, 5 g); Protein, 26g; Fat, 29g (suitable for all phases)

Cottage Cheese with Vanilla, Pistachio Nuts, Cinnamon, and Orange Zest or Marmalade

I also eat this for dessert. Tastes like cheesecake if you squint.

6 ounces cottage cheese (I used full-fat to calculate nutrition), 1 ounce dry-roasted salted pistachios, dash cinnamon, ¼ teaspoon orange zest, ½ tablespoon marmalade (or your favorite jelly), plus splash of vanilla extract. Skip the marmalade if you want to follow a stricter keto program.

361 Calories; Carb, 23g (Fiber, 4g); Protein, 28 g; Fat, 21 g (suitable for all phases)

Hawaiian Dream: Mango Mac-Nut Dairy Fusion

This special parfait was inspired by foraging through gift snacks patients on Kauai brought from their yards to my office.

6 ounces Greek yogurt (no-fat since it's higher in protein and we're adding high-fat ingredients), 1 ounce macadamia nuts, 2 tablespoons finely chopped dried mango, 2 ounces full-fat coconut milk, ½ ounce watermelon seeds, ¼ teaspoon minced ginger.
530 Calories; Carb, 26 g (Fiber, 3 g); Protein, 27 g; Fat, 27 g (suitable for all phases)

YOGURT AND CHIA PUDDING TOPPING COMBOS FOR PHASE I BREAKFAST AND LUNCH

You can experiment with combinations of your favorite nuts, seeds, spices, and fruits to dress up plain regular or Greek yogurt and chia puddings. Here, I've given you my favorite combinations.

Use as much of the nuts, seeds, and spices as you like. Use 1 to 2 teaspoons of dried fruit and 2 to 3 tablespoons of fresh to keep the sugar content under control.

Cinnamon Raisin: Wheat germ, raisins, cinnamon
Apple Walnut: Walnut pieces, shredded apple, cinnamon
Pecan Pie: Roasted salted pecans, wheat germ, pecan pie spices (ground cloves, anise seeds, cinnamon), and ½ to 1 teaspoon maple syrup or honey
Mandarin Pistachio: Salted roasted pistachio, mandarin orange wedge, unsweetened shredded coconut or coconut flakes (2 tablespoons)

WHAT ELSE CAN I EAT FOR LUNCH?

Any lunch that is vegetable-oil-free, gives you plenty of good fats, and has less than 30 grams of net carbohydrate will help keep your energy up all afternoon. Keep in mind that your daily carb total in the baby steps part of Phase I should always be 100 grams or less, and ideally 75 or less.

PHASE I DINNER IDEAS

The main goal during Phase I is to learn to adapt whatever you usually make for dinner so that it's in alignment with the big five rules. As with breakfast and lunch, you'll be using healthy fats and plenty of salt. And you'll be learning to cut down on starchy carbs like rice, bread, noodles, and potatoes, or swap them out for slow-digesting carbs to keep you full so that you don't feel you have to fill up on after-dinner snacks.

Side dishes can be changed easily since they're not integral to the meal. Common starchy carb-rich dinnertime sides include bread (except sprouted grain breads—those are OK), rice, and potatoes. A super simple swap-out for starch/carbs could include broccoli, string beans, garden peas, Brussels sprouts, or spinach. All of those taste great steamed with plenty of garlic butter and salt.

For starchy carbs that are usually part of the meal, like pasta and rice, use the chart on page 246 to find an alternative.

For entrées, you can keep your usual routines with meats, fish, eggs, and vegetables, while being sure to include plenty of clean-burning fats. Clean-burning fats are especially helpful when you use lean meats like chicken breast, tuna, 95 percent lean ground beef, and well-trimmed steaks. If you don't usually include healthy fats with your leaner meats, you can include them with your veggies instead. If you find yourself hungry for second helpings of your meat and veggies, adding more healthy fats next time will help.

THE CARB-SWAP DINNER TRANSFORMATION GAME

Here are some swap-out examples to help you transform recipes you already make.

Swap-Out Chart

STARCHY CARB	SLOW CARB
PASTA	Spiralized ZUCCHINI ("Zoodles") Spiralized BUTTERNUT SQUASH **BEAN-Based Pasta **CHICKPEA-Based Pasta (**e.g. *Explore Cuisine***)
RICE	WILD RICE CAULIFLOWER RICE SHREDDED CABBAGE ZOODLES BEANS
BREAD	SPROUTED GRAIN BREAD SOURDOUGH BREAD (MAX 1 SLICE)
POTATOES	BEANS CAULIFLOWER RICE SHREDDED CABBAGE

Use the swap-out chart for ideas on making the same dishes you already make a lot healthier. For soups that might include potatoes, try beans instead. Great northern and cannellini are mild-tasting substitutes. If the soup includes rice, try riced cauliflower. For casseroles that might include pasta, try one of the bean-based pasta brands, or zucchini slices or zucchini noodles.

Let's go over a few specific examples of upgraded dinners you can make simply by swapping out starchy carb for slow carb.

Meat and Potatoes

Say you normally cook your family juicy steaks with baked potatoes, bread, and green peas for dinner. If your family is not joining you in your

PHASE I SAMPLE DINNER SWAP-OUTS

INSTEAD OF THIS	TRY THIS
Pasta with Sauce	LESS PASTA with UPGRADED SAUCE
Taco Tuesday!	UPGRADED TACO TUESDAY
Burgers and Dogs	BUNLESS BURGERS and RECONSTRUCTED CORN DOGS
Microwave Dinner	UPGRADED MICROWAVE DINNERS
No Veggies	FROZEN VEGGIES
Baked Potato	ROASTED VEGGIES
Store-Bought Salad Dressing	BASIC SALAD DRESSING: QUALITY OIL AND VINEGAR

efforts to get healthy, feed them as usual, but for you, skip the bread, give yourself a bigger portion of the greens, and either skip the baked potato or cut it in half, while making sure to add plenty of clean-burning fat-rich fixings like butter, sour cream, bacon, and melted cheese.

Less Pasta with Upgraded Sauce

Say you normally cook pasta with meat sauce, bread, and salad. If you're not ready for spiralized zucchini or other pasta substitutes, you can simply use less pasta and make up the volume difference by adding more veggies and more meat to your pasta sauce to create a super sauce. Use more of everything except the tomato paste: extra meat, plenty of mushrooms, onion, and green bell peppers. I use about two pounds of meat in my meat sauce, with massive amounts of veggies, and top with plenty of parmesan cheese. I actually do not use any pasta at all anymore since I don't want to "water down" the yummy sauce.

If you're starting with a jar sauce, make sure to read ingredients to avoid the three C and three S vegetable oils. A small minority of brands use olive oil. Right now Ragú makes a line using only olive oil and no junk oils called Simply Chunky, as does Rao's. But check the label every time you buy, as companies can change ingredients at any time.

Upgraded Taco Tuesday!

Instead of hard taco shells, which are loaded with toxic oils, use yellow corn masa tortillas. There are many brands available at local grocery stores. Mission and La Tortilla Factory are easy to find. To reduce the relative carbohydrate content and thereby make "space" in your calorie budget for the higher-fat toppings, instead of using the shell like a pocket, use it like pizza dough and pile the meat and toppings in a nice big heap, then eat with knife and fork.

Boneless Burgers and Reconstructed Corn Dogs

Hot dogs and burgers are great without the buns—or you can just use half a bun at first (I'll give you a full recipe for burgers in Chapter 13). Get creative with your toppings. Try different cheeses, sun-dried tomatoes, mustards, and condiments. Skip the fries and go for oven-roasted veggies—you'll find yourself getting a lot more flavor.

Reconstructed Corn Dog

Use a 6-inch corn tortilla and 2 ounces cheddar cheese; melt (on high in the microwave for 35 seconds), then add 2 ounces deli-sliced ham or a grass-fed hot dog (presliced on the diagonal to be fancy) and heat for another 20 seconds or so to warm the meat. Then add a schmear of mustard and 1 to 2 ounces sauerkraut. Ham version: 370 Calories; Carb, 15 g (Fiber, 2 g); Protein, 27 g; Fat, 23 g.

Upgraded Microwave Dinners

Instead of buying frozen microwavable dinners, try frozen ingredients and heat them together in a casserole dish in a microwave, covered. Here's a couple ideas to get you thinking:

- Chicken + broccoli florets + zucchini + cheddar cheese + butter + garlic powder + onion powder + salt

- Meatballs + sliced bell peppers and stir-fry veggies + sweet-and-sour sauce + garlic powder + soy sauce (sparingly)

Frozen Veggies, Warmed and Sautéed

Frozen veggies can have anywhere from roughly equal to significantly less nutrition than fresh—it all depends on how long they've been in the freezer. That said, they are going to be better than canned because they have not been heated to death, simply flash-cooked before being flash-frozen. And frozen veggies are far healthier than potato, rice, or bread-based sides.

You can cook frozen veggies in a microwave, but if you have access to a stovetop and a decent pan, you can heat the veggies through in some butter nearly as quickly as you could heat them in a microwave and they will taste ten times better.

The best low-carb frozen veggies, flavor-wise, for pan frying will be:

- Green peas (baby and regular-size)
- Green beans, not French cut (they get freezer burned more easily)
- Edamame (shell removed)—these go great with fresh cherry tomatoes, halved and slathered in fish and soy sauce
- Lima beans—these taste best when you fry them in unsalted butter until their outer skin shrivels, then salt
- Spinach—needs garlic butter (a lot) or a roux, cream, and nutmeg (see mac and cheese recipe on page 306 for making a roux)
- Bell peppers—these taste best when you use them in a stir-fry
- Mushrooms—also best with a stir-fry

Frozen Peas

Pour the amount of peas you want in a pot without any butter. Turn on high and stay nearby so you can listen for the sound of the water sizzling. Stir until the sizzle stops, just a few seconds. Every 30 seconds or so stir again. After the peas are no longer frosty, add 1 to 2 pats of butter per cup of peas, stir to get that butter down in the heat, and then cover your pot, remove from heat, and let sit for 2 to 4 minutes until butter is melted.

Roasted Veggies

Roasted vegetables are universally pleasurable to eat. Cut to uniform sizes, coat with olive oil, salt and pepper, and place on a tray large enough to give vegetables their own space (so they dry) and cook in a hot oven for an appropriate amount of time.

Basic Salad Dressing: Quality Oil and Vinegar

Use 1 to 2 tablespoons olive, peanut, or sesame oil per person plus ½ to 1 teaspoon clear vinegar or balsamic, which goes best with olive oil. Sprinkle salt liberally. For just one or two people it's often easier to pour over each bowl rather than make up a big batch.

For more flavor use garlic powder, parmesan, or your favorite herb mix.

A short cut for flavor if you're not good with herbs and spices is to buy seasoning mixes and sprinkle over your salad. Hidden Valley is available everywhere, and they have a wide range of choices. Spice mixes often contain bad oils to help prevent caking, but the amount is generally low and not worth worrying about.

For additional dressing recipes, see Chapters 13 and 14.

WHAT ELSE CAN I EAT FOR DINNER?

Any dinner that is vegetable-oil-free, gives you plenty of good fats and whole food proteins, and has less than 50 grams of net carbohydrate (including beverages and desserts) will send you off to dreamland in good shape.

STOCKING YOUR KITCHEN: PHASE I/BEGINNER

I recommend you phase out any foods containing vegetable oils, including snacks, condiments, frozen foods, and ready-to-eat foods.

I don't recommend throwing away any raw ingredients except the vegetable oils. So you can keep flour, sugar, honey, maple syrup, and so on. I do recommend using these blood-sugar-raising ingredients a lot less than most people currently do.

SHOPPING LIST FOR PHASE I

The idea of the plan is to help folks make most of their dinners in thirty minutes or less and most breakfasts and lunches in ten minutes or less. Therefore, these are ingredients you can use to make those kinds of meals. If you already are good at making meals that take more time, like roasts and slow-cooked or braised dishes, then by all means keep doing those.

Assuming a few basics, like sugar, flour, baking soda, and so on that most people have, I've listed a few essential items that you will want to consider for this phase to start rebuilding your healthy kitchen. You will be using these items in the next phase as well. The following are intended to help out the kitchen novice and are not at all exhaustive recommendations. Those who are experienced cooks will probably want to keep much more variety on hand.

Pantry Items

Fats and oils: Choose at least three fats and oils from the good fats list on page 223

Vinegar: Choose at least one: apple cider, balsamic, rice, white, wine

Basic condiments: Avocado oil mayo, hot sauce, ketchup (with 5 grams sugar or less per serving), mustard (yellow, Dijon—all the basic mustard styles I've seen are good), soy sauce, tabasco, seasonings, herbs, and spices: In addition to salt and black pepper, I suggest you choose three or four from at least three of your favorite culinary regions to make sure you've got a good choice of compatible spices. For example, Mediterranean: garlic powder, Italian seasoning mix, bay leaf, basil; Mexican: cumin, chili powder, Mexican oregano, onion powder. Indian: curry powder, ginger powder, cinnamon, coriander.

Ready-to-Eat

Corn masa tortilla: Store in your fridge once opened.

Nuts: At least two of your favorites, raw or dry-roasted (no vegetable oil); salted is fine.

Seeds: Raw or sprouted pumpkin or sunflower seeds (they are delicious sprouted).

Canned and Jarred Goods

Beans (one or two kinds), canned tomatoes, jelly (less than 7 grams sugar per tablespoon), olives (green, black, or kalamata), no-vegetable-oil-added peanut butter (or any nut butter), sun-dried tomatoes

Chicken stock (made with bones)

Salmon (canned, bone-in gives you extra calcium)

Tuna (canned in water or olive oil to avoid the vegetable oils; salt is fine)

Chill

Dairy: Butter, cheese, half-and-half or cream, and yogurt are essentials. If you are lactose-intolerant, choose fermented cheeses that are naturally lactose-free like cheddar, provolone, Muenster, and Swiss. Many fermented yogurts are also naturally low in lactose.

Eggs: Buy at least a dozen—they keep for weeks.

Sprouted grain bread: Store in your fridge, or the freezer if you use less than one loaf every two weeks.

Very perishable basic veggies: Buy at least two each week of the following beginner veggies: bell peppers, lettuces (like arugula, romaine), salad-green and baby-green tubs, fresh herbs (basil, cilantro).

Less perishable basic veggies: Always have at least two on hand: asparagus, broccoli, Brussels sprouts, cabbage, cauliflower, celery, kale, radish, string beans.

Least perishable basic veggies: Carrots, garlic, ginger root, onions.

Frozen basic veggies: Keep at least one of these in your freezer at all times for emergency greens: green peas, spinach, green beans, broccoli.

Basic ready-to-eat meats: Buy at least two of each of the following each week: nitrate-free deli meats, nitrate-free precooked sausage, nitrate-free grass-fed hot dogs.

Frozen, precooked but unseasoned (to avoid vegetable oil): Chicken.

Basic meats: Buy at least two of each of the following each week (plan on using about 2 to 3 pounds of fresh meat per person per week): Bacon; chicken legs, wings, and breasts; fresh pork sausage, no casing; ground beef or chicken; steak (beef, lamb steaks, or pork chops); turkey breast or ground turkey.

13

Phase I

Metabolic Rehab: The Accelerated Plan

IN THIS CHAPTER YOU'LL LEARN TO

- Use keto recipes to accelerate your metabolic rehab.
- Enjoy carbs while experiencing keto benefits.
- Find fast easy recipes with Google and YouTube.

In the last chapter, the goal was to get started becoming your new, healthiest self by adding new, healthy habits at your own pace. You are ready to consider the accelerated steps if you feel you have mastered the five rules, have stopped snacking, and have no hypoglycemia. In other words, once you're down to just three meals a day and feeling fine, then you're ready to boost your metabolic recovery by using the meal-planning ideas and recipes in this chapter.

The boost comes from a focus on following something like a keto diet by day and having the option of continuing keto at dinnertime or including a few slow-digesting carbs. You'll be including more of the clean-burning fats that can help accelerate the process of gaining control over sugar and carb cravings.

ACCELERATED GOALS

Your goal during this phase is to smash your hunger with clean-burning fats. Formulating your breakfast, lunch, and dinner around the five rules, you may find that you go for days without feeling the slightest hunger twinge. Now you're ready for keto.

The metabolic rehabilitation effect of a keto-style diet comes from the abundance of clean-burning fats and relative absence of anything that could jack up your insulin. The presence of energy-boosting fat helps to train your brain to "trust" fat again, and to give up its love affair with sugar. Eating healthy, hunger-suppressing fats is the best way to retrain your carb-addicted brain to stop obsessing about starchy, sweet, and otherwise carb-loaded foods. The absence of insulin helps free fat from storage between meals. As your metabolism makes repairs, you'll shift from burning the calories in your last meal to burning your own body fat.

To accelerate your fatburn, you'll need to consume no more than 50 grams of carbohydrate per day. And remember, the time of day you eat those carbs makes a huge difference. Thanks to the morning cortisol pulse and your daytime activity, the worst time to include carbs is with breakfast and the best time to get those carbohydrates is with dinner—as we learned in Chapter 6 (Fatburn System 2: Hormones That Control Blood Sugar).

If you're feeling intimidated by the idea of counting up every gram of carb in all your meals, don't be. I find that most folks don't actually have to go through the trouble unless they run into a road block. And the road blocks usually happen for one of two easily remedied reasons for overeating. First, you are still so hungry at meals that you take overly large portions. This is usually happening because, in the meal prior to the one you're overeating, you didn't get enough fat. Second, you're in the habit of filling up on carbs and now you want to eat the same volume of higher-calories foods. You can't.

KETO BY DAY

I've talked a bit about ketones, but not about the keto diet itself. Because you'll be following something like a keto diet if you opt into this accelerated portion of Phase I, let's discuss the diet in a little more detail.

The ketogenic diet, "keto" for short, is a diet that's low in carbohydrate and high in fat, similar to the Atkins diet. Unlike most other low-carb diets, the keto diet is the only popular diet that specifically instructs you to seek out foods containing plenty of those clean-burning fats. I believe the healthy fats, and not the lack of carbs, is the reason the keto diet is one of the most effective popular diets in history. In directing you to eat more foods like butter, eggs, avocados, and nuts, while avoiding chips and junk foods loaded with toxic fats, it's helping folks follow the number one most important fatburn rule: "Avoid vegetable oil."

Despite the name, you won't be eating ketones on a keto diet because there are no foods that contain ketones. No part of your body is made of ketones, either. The diet gets its name from the fact that you are supporting your body's ability to *generate* ketones. You accelerate your fatburn by cutting your carbs as if you were following a keto diet during the daytime. At night, however, there will still be room for some slow carbs if you want to include these, as we have discussed.

Just because you're following a keto-style diet, that doesn't mean that your body will immediately start pumping out ketones. While cutting carbs is essential to repairing your metabolism, you may not be able to produce much in the way of ketones until Phase II, when you start restricting calories. That's totally fine, because the goal of the Phase I accelerated metabolic rehabilitation is not to produce ketones. The goal is to prepare your body's fatburning systems so that when you start restricting calories, you feel fantastic thanks to the fact that you can finally burn your body fat.

HOW MUCH CARB IS TOO MUCH CARB FOR KETO?

In this accelerated metabolic rehabilitation portion of Phase I, we're going for keto or nearly keto macros. This is the only time I'll ask you to pay close attention to your carb intake. To get the benefits of keto, you need to keep your total daily carb counts between 20 and 50 grams. Your breakfast should contain the least amount of carb, and dinner the most. I recommend the following carb ranges for each meal: breakfast, 0 to 15 grams; lunch, 0 to 30 grams; and dinner, 0 to 50 grams.

You may have read lower numbers elsewhere. Dr. Atkins, the original guru of the keto diet, recommended no more than 20 grams of carb per day for optimal ketone production. But I suggest you don't need to be that strict all the time, which is why I allow up to 50 grams. The problem with this 20-grams-or-bust line of thinking is it overlooks other factors that influence your body's ketone production.

First, if your metabolism is very unhealthy, ketosis may not benefit you at all because burning body fat releases the same kinds of fatty acids that caused all your problems in the first place, which deepens your metabolic problems. Second, the typical keto plan allows people to snack as often as they like. Snacking on anything—even high-fat foods—often stops ketone production. Third, the typical keto plan does not discriminate between carb in the morning, when it blocks fatburn most powerfully, and carb at the end of the day, when it blocks fatburn least powerfully. Finally, the typical keto plan does not distinguish between slow-digesting carbs and big piles of starchy carb and sugars.

In my view, sustaining the more extreme low-carbohydrate intake of 20 grams day after day is simply not necessary. In my view, the end goal is not to produce ketones. The end goal is to improve your metabolic health and fatburn. A near-keto diet does the job without the extreme dietary restriction that makes people feel bad if they have a slice of quality pizza, or even the occasional beer.

KETO-Compatible WHOLE FOOD List

ANIMAL-BASED FOODS

Low-carb dairy: Milk, yogurt, cottage cheese, goat cheese, ricotta
Low-carb seafood: Oysters, mussels, abalone, whelk

You can enjoy these low-carb dairy and seafoods on a keto diet, but don't make them the foundation of multiple meals.

Zero-carb: Eggs; land-animal muscle meats; poultry; organ meats; tuna, salmon, and other fish

PLANT-BASED FOODS

Most plant-based foods will contain carbs, including fiber. Animal products do not contain fiber, while there are many kinds of "fiber" in plants. Some kinds of fiber break down into sugar, while others do not. The nutrition label does not tell you how much of each is present in the food, leaving us to guess. If you're counting your carbs, most folks advise that you subtract half the fiber grams from the total carb count to estimate the amount of sugar that enters the bloodstream. So for example if we're looking at peanut butter with 6 grams of total carb and 2 grams of fiber per serving, then you can subtract one of those fiber grams, leaving your intake at 5 grams.

NUTS AND SEEDS

Higher-carb content: Cashews, pistachios, pumpkin seeds
You can enjoy higher-carb nuts and seeds on a keto diet, but don't add more than 1 to 2 ounces to multiple meals.
Lower-carb content: Almonds, Brazil nuts, chia seeds, hemp hearts, macadamia nuts, pecans, peanuts, poppy seeds, sesame seeds, sunflower seeds, walnuts, hazelnuts, pine nuts

VEGGIES

Veggies vary greatly in their carb content. I've broken them into four broad categories: starchy, semi-starchy, low-carb, and nearly carb-free.

Starchy veggies (avoid in Phase I Accelerated): Potatoes, rice (1 cup cooked = about 30+ g)
Semi-starchy veggies (max 1 cup/day in Phase I Accelerated): Corn, peas, winter squashes, beans (pinto, soy, kidney, garbanzo, etc.) (1 cup cooked = about 20–30 g)
Low-carb veggies (max 2 cups/day in Phase I Accelerated): Beets, bell pepper, cabbage, cauliflower, broccoli, Brussels sprouts, carrots, sprouts, onion, spring peas, summer squashes, string beans, turnip, zucchini (1 cup = about 10–20 g)
Nearly carb-free veggies (hard to overeat these): Green onion; leafy greens like kale, spinach, baby greens, and lettuce; bean sprouts like mung beans and lentil sprouts; bitter-tasting veggies like

celery and radish; all herbs and spices; mushrooms (1 cup = less than 10 g)

What's Included?

As in Chapter 12, I'm not going to fill this chapter with a lot of detailed recipes for dishes you may or may not even end up liking. Instead, I'm going to give you easy-to-read tables of ideas on how to take advantage of the many keto-friendly recipes on the web. I'll also give you more detailed instructions for just a few essential recipes and introduce you to a few essential skills that will help you master the art of making fast, healthy meals.

PHASE I ACCELERATED BREAKFAST IDEAS

Popular keto-style breakfast options provide plenty of healthy fat and over-all less carb than Phase I options. These options are also suitable for Phase I, though keto all day is not recommended during Phase I.

PHASE I ACCELERATED BREAKFAST MENU	
EGGS 101 WAYS	• 1-3 eggs, 1-2 Tbsp cooking fat, optional bacon/sausage/herbs/veg
KETO CHIA BOWL	• Same as Phase I but less fruit or no fruit
KETO YOGURT PARFAIT	• Same as Phase I but less fruit or no fruit
KETO BREAKFAST SMOOTHIE	• Same as Phase I but less fruit or no fruit
SPROUTED GRAIN TOAST	• 1 slice toast loaded with savory toppings
BULLETPROOF COFFEE	• Same as Phase I
HIGH-OCTANE MILK	• Cow's milk or almond milk with additional fat of choice
HERBAL TEA UNSWEETENED	• Any herbal tea without sweetener

Eggs 101 Ways

Eggs make a super healthy breakfast. Use one to three eggs poached, hard boiled, scrambled, sunny side up, or any way you like, and include any of the non-starchy veggies you like.

Keto Chia Bowl

Follow the same instructions as in the last chapter to make the chia pudding base. For toppings that are keto compatible (lower in carb and higher in fat), use the guidelines in Topping Combos for Phase I Accelerated (page 266). It's easy to find keto-compatible recipes on Google and YouTube, so go crazy! Many recipes use artificial sweeteners that you can skip or try to use the smallest amount you need.

Keto Yogurt Parfait

Follow the same instructions as in the Baby Steps for the yogurt itself. Use the guidelines in Topping Combos for Phase I Accelerated (page 266). If you cannot find whole milk Greek or regular yogurt, be sure to add sour cream, crème fraîche, whipped cream (no sugar added), coconut cream, or use plenty of very high fat toppings.

Keto Breakfast Smoothie

Follow the same instructions as for Phase I, but use only ¼ cup fresh melon or berries, like strawberries, raspberries, or blueberries, or go fruit-free. Do a Google or YouTube search for "Keto smoothie" for more ideas.

Bulletproof Coffee

Bulletproof coffee is low in carb and high enough in fat so that the same instructions as in the last chapter are suitable for the Accelerated Plan.

Sprouted Grain Toast

See Chapter 12.

High-Octane Milk

1 cup milk (almond, soy, or cow's) plus additional ⅛ cup of dairy cream, coconut cream, and optional vanilla extract and cinnamon or nutmeg sprinkle.

Herbal Tea Unsweetened (Ideally)

Same as in the previous chapter, but try to see if you like it without the sweetener. Stevia drops would be OK if you really prefer it with a sweetener.

WHAT ELSE CAN I EAT FOR BREAKFAST?

Any breakfast that is vegetable-oil-free, gives you plenty of good fats, and has 10 grams or fewer of net carbohydrate will help keep your energy up all morning long.

PHASE I ACCELERATED LUNCH IDEAS

These lunch ideas are all similar to breakfast: no toxic oils, plenty of healthy fat, a little slow-digesting carb, and whole food protein. The difference between the last chapter and this accelerated portion of Phase I is that here we're going for keto or nearly keto macros. For lunch we're going for no more than 20 grams of carb, and lower is better.

Popular keto-style lunch options provide plenty of healthy fat and overall less carb than Phase I options. See the Phase I Accelerated Lunch Menu on page 341 (at the end of the Resources section).

Lunch Option Details

Tuna or Egg Salad (No Bread)

I can tuna (in olive oil or water to avoid vegetable oils) dressed with:

CHEF DEBBIE LEE'S SESAME DIJON DRESSING

2 tablespoons toasted sesame oil

I teaspoon Dijon mustard

I teaspoon rice vinegar (or apple cider or white vinegar)

I teaspoon soy sauce or tamari

Or 2 to 3 hard-boiled eggs, sliced (an egg slicer makes this easier) and dressed with:

E-Z EGG SALAD DRESSING

  2 tablespoons mayo (check label to make sure no C or S oils)

  I teaspoon Dijon mustard

  I teaspoon sweet pickle relish or I tablespoon finely chopped celery plus
  squirt of lemon juice

  Salt to taste

Mason Jar Salads

Pack these in one-quart, glass mason jars to bring to work or on the road. Keep chilled in insulated bags. It's easy to find recipes for these that use what you've got in the fridge; just google the phrase "low-carb mason jar salad" or "keto mason jar salad" in quotes, plus the ingredient you need to use (cucumber, cauliflower, etc.). The same process works to find videos on YouTube. These are a couple to get you going.

Roast Chicken Pecan Prosciutto and Brie Bites Spinach Salad

  2 teaspoons pepper jelly

  ½ tablespoon olive oil

  2 ounces leftover or deli-sliced chicken

  ½ teaspoon apple cider or balsamic vinegar

  I cup fresh baby spinach leaves

  I ounce Brie cheese cubed

  ½ ounce prosciutto cut into I-inch strips

  I ounce roasted salted pecans

500 Calories; Carb, 19g (Fiber, 4g); Protein, 27g; Fat, 35g

1. Mix the pepper jelly into the olive oil for consistency. A serrated butter knife cuts Brie better than a sharp knife.

2. Bring to work in a mason jar by layering the bottom with chicken, then add oil-and-jelly mix and vinegar (to marinate chicken), then layer spinach over that, layer Brie and prosciutto over the spinach, and top with pecans to maintain crunch.

3. To make for a satisfying dinner, double the spinach and meat, and ratchet up the other ingredients a notch.

Peanut-y Thai Chicken with Romaine

You don't need to go to a restaurant to enjoy the exotic flavors of Thailand. Just invest in sriracha and combine with peanuts and lime.

1 tablespoon peanut butter
½ tablespoon olive oil
¼ cup sliced or shredded carrot
2 tablespoons chopped red onion
½ teaspoon lime juice or vinegar
2 ounces rotisserie or other leftover chicken (or deli slices)
¼ cup cucumber slices
½ cup chopped or torn romaine lettuce
½ teaspoon sriracha a.k.a. rooster sauce
310 Calories; Carb, 10g (Fiber, 3g); Protein, 15g; Fat, 24g

1. Mix the peanut butter with the olive oil for better consistency.
2. Bring to work in a mason jar by layering the bottom with carrots and red onion, then add lime juice to marinate the veggies, then add chicken and apply the oil-and-peanut-butter mix, then cucumber slices and romaine. Sprinkle on the sriracha.
3. To make for a satisfying dinner, double the veggies and meat and ratchet up the other ingredients a notch.

Wrap 'n' Roll

Deli wraps will make you confident that a "sandwich" can be great even if you shed the bread. Here are a few popular combinations to get you started, and I encourage you to try your hand at experimenting with new ideas using your favorite meats, veggies, cheese, and condiments.

Salami, Cream Cheese, and Herb Baked String Beans

Whole fresh string beans baked with herbs, wrap 2 or 3 at a time together with 1 slice of nitrate-free salami that you've smeared with a small amount of cream cheese, or garlic-and-herb cream cheese you've whipped ahead—total 2 tablespoons cream cheese; then, since the salami can "sweat" at room

temperature, use 1 thin-sliced baked chicken deli slice as the outermost wrap. Six rolls should fill you up. Don't slice these as they'll fall apart.
400 Calories; Carb, 13g (Fiber, 3g); Protein, 26g; Fat, 29g

Ham-It-Up Dill Pickles

Take 2 to 3 pieces of thinly sliced ham (depending on size of pickle), and place them on a cutting board overlapping half of each with the next. Spread 1 ounce cream cheese (herbed cream cheese, or blend in a few shakes from a packet of ranch dressing mix) onto each strip of meat, then wrap around your dill pickle. Use a total of 4 ounces meat, 2 to 3 pickles, and 2 ounces cream cheese. Other meats that work with this idea are salami or any dried beef product. Slice into ½- to ¾-inch pieces.
400 Calories (for ham edition); Carb, 10g (Fiber, 3g); Protein, 23g; Fat, 30g

Turkey and Swiss

This is my favorite—no spread required, just good-tasting main ingredients.

Start with ¼ pound of deli-sliced turkey and 2½ or so ounces of thin-sliced deli-style Swiss cheese. Combine 2 to 3 slices of turkey with each slice of Swiss cheese. Add mustard or horseradish, optionally. Roll into romaine lettuce and slice into pinwheels.
400 Calories; Carb, 10g (Fiber, 0g); Protein, 32g; Fat, 25g

Popular Pinwheels

You can also wrap any of the above with a collard, romaine, or kale leaf. When working with collard and kale, use a sharp knife to thin the stem, carving off some of the width of the stem as you move up the leaf so that the leaf flexes more easily. Wrapping tightly makes it easier to slice into an attractive pinwheel that will impress your friends.

Other Tasty Deli-Meat-and-Cheese Combinations

- Provolone cheese and roast beef (optional horseradish and mayo)

- Salami and provolone (optional pepperoncini and chopped onion)
- Ham and Swiss (optional mustard and mayo)
- Capocollo and mozzarella (optional basil leaves or pine nut pesto)

Melts in Your Mouth

Place pieces of your favorite cheese on a large plate, then melt on high for 15 seconds in the microwave before wrapping the thinnest slice of meat around the molten blob. This is a great variation and you don't need any condiments. I go to Costco and get some of their fancy hard cheeses to combine with their higher-end deli meat.

Do-It-Yourself Instant Soups

If you start with a good stock or broth and add a few flavorful ingredients, you can make a fast, healthy lunch in 5 to 15 minutes. A couple ideas that work great with just a little planning ahead:

Sesame Ginger Chicken 'n' Egg (single serving, 15 minutes)

Sauté a quarter of an onion, diced, in 1 tablespoon butter until soft. Add 2 cups of chicken broth and bring to a boil. While waiting, taste and add salt as needed. Once the water is boiling, turn heat to medium low, add 1 teaspoon ground ginger and 1 tablespoon sesame oil, then slowly drop in 2 eggs to poach for 2 to 3 minutes until desired doneness.

Curried Kale and Sausage (single serving, 5 minutes)

Heat 2 cups of your favorite chicken stock or broth in a saucepan. Add 2 cups of chopped kale, 1 precooked sausage, sliced, and 1 teaspoon of your favorite curry powder. After the kale is cooked and sausage is hot throughout, add 1 tablespoon cream to finish.

Keto-Crust Pizza

Major chains like Costco and Walmart now carry some version of cauliflower pizza crust. You just need to add your toppings and sauce. Makes a great dinner when you load it up with precooked ground beef or sausage.

TOPPING COMBOS FOR PHASE I ACCELERATED BREAKFAST AND LUNCH

These additional combinations of nuts, fruits, spices, and so on also work well as toppings for yogurt or chia pudding. Use as much of the nuts, seeds, and spices as you like.

Almond Joy

½ to 1 ounce almonds, 2 drops almond extract (optional), 1 to 2 tablespoons cacao nibs, 2 tablespoons shredded or flaked coconut

Fennel and Cinnamon

Sprouted pumpkin seeds, shredded coconut or coconut flakes (unsweetened), fennel seeds (½ to 1 teaspoon per serving), cinnamon or cinnamon spice mix (⅛ teaspoon), hemp seeds (1 tablespoon)

Orange Ginger

Pistachio, shredded coconut or coconut flakes (unsweetened), candied ginger slices minced finely, orange zest

Peaches and Cream

Almonds, sour cream, hemp hearts, toasted wheat germ, 4 to 8 drops Bakto Natural Peach Flavor (made with all-natural essences and extracts)

Jelly Vanilly

Your favorite jam or jelly (better-quality jams have 7 grams or less sugar per tablespoon), vanilla extract, pistachio nuts dusted with cinnamon powder

WHAT ELSE CAN I EAT FOR LUNCH?

Any lunch that is vegetable-oil-free and contains less than 20 gram of net carb will help sustain your energy all afternoon. Keep in mind, to accelerate your metabolic recovery, your daily carb total should always be 50 grams or less, and some days should be even lower—as low as you can go.

#GOALS: FIND NEW FOODS YOU LOVE

I do not expect you to eat foods you don't enjoy. If you try any of these foods and find you really don't like them, then I want you to try something else. I really don't want you to buy into the idea that you should force yourself to eat something you don't like just because it's healthy for you.

For this to be sustainable, we need to find foods that you love. Real ingredients have good taste. You don't have to like every food on earth—I know I don't, and I'm convinced we'll find plenty of real ingredients that you like.

The key is learning to combine flavors, and the recipes included offer you a lot of ideas on what flavors tend to go together. You may not like tomatoes in a salad for example, but love them in salsa where they're combined with salt, garlic, cilantro, onion, and other flavorful ingredients. Or you may not like broccoli, but you've never tried it slathered in garlic butter and salt. Very often when I work with chefs, they tell me that their clients who are sure they hate certain foods have enjoyed them over and over in the dishes they make, sometimes without even knowing it.

PHASE I ACCELERATED DINNER IDEAS

As you know, we're going for keto or nearly keto macros, and this is the only Phase where I'll ask you to pay close attention to your carb intake. You can enjoy relatively more carb at dinner, but your daily total must remain under 50 to get the benefits of this Accelerated Plan. What you can eat at dinner to experience those benefits therefore depends on what you ate during the rest of the day. If you had a zero-carb egg and bacon breakfast, another zero-carb wrap and roll for lunch, then for dinner you could max it out at 50 grams. Of course you can also eat less.

Remember, if you have gotten used to cooking lean meat, like chicken, you definitely need to be sure to include a high-fat sauce or side. One simple tip to getting plenty of fat is to eat more veggies with butter, cream, or cheese sauces.

These popular keto-style dinner options provide plenty of healthy fat and overall less carb than Phase I Baby Steps options. There are thousands more ideas and detailed recipes available to you, but these are a few that are superfast and simple to give you ideas and get you started on your way.

PHASE I ACCELERATED DINNER MENU
ASTERISK INDICATES RECIPE INCLUDED

ROTISSERIE OR AIR FRYER CHICKEN	• Buy grocery store rotisserie or use an air fryer
STIR FRY 'N' VEGGIES (no rice)	• Fill your family up with rice if they insist, keep the veggies to yourself
ZOODLES WITH UPGRADED SAUCE	• Spiralized zucchini makes a great pasta substitute
KETO CASSEROLE	• 5 ingredients or less, bakes in 30 minutes
BARE NAKED BURGER & SALAD*	• Burgers cook while you chop up salad
SOUP IS GOOD FOOD	• Soup up any soup by substituting beans for rice or potatoes and adding ample veggies
STEAMED VEGGIES in GARLIC BUTTER*	• If you like garlic bread, you'll love these no-guilt garlic butter veggies
THE LAND OF SALAD*	• Salad side and salad main courses with zero cooking required

DINNER OPTION DETAILS

Rotisserie or Air Fryer Chicken

Most grocery stores make and sell ready-to-eat slow-cooked rotisserie chicken. This is a great easy option for the day you do your grocery shopping or even to serve as a substitute for takeout. While you're at the store, you can buy some fresh veggies for a salad or steamed side. (See "Steamed Broccoli," page 273, for instructions on how to steam veggies.) When cooking at home, air frying works best for skin-on chicken legs, wings, and thighs. Air fryer recipes are easy to find on the web, but all you need is a simple coat of olive or peanut oil about two-thirds of the way through the cooking process along with your favorite spice rub—you can even just use salt and pepper.

Stir-Fry 'n' Veggies (no rice)

Stir-fries are simply vegetables and proteins fried quickly in flavorful oils and sauces. They are super healthy, super flexible, and only require one cooking container—a wok, or a regular large flat-bottom fry pan. You can use the tougher, cheaper cuts of beef and pork that would ordinarily require roasting or slow cooking if you slice the meat thin and marinate it for a minimum of an hour (and up to twenty-four hours) ahead.

Stir-frying is all about the prep, meaning slicing your protein and veggies ahead of time, and having your oils, sauces, and spices nearby. Plan for the prep to take 10 to 20 minutes and the cooking time 5 to 15, depending on how many portions you are making.

You don't need any rice to enjoy stir-fry. Skipping the rice saves you time and allows you to focus on the more nutritious vegetables and proteins instead. If you do want rice, be sure to limit it to ½ to ¾ cup per serving, or just enough to sop up any additional sauce.

There are just a few essential rules to ensure stir-fry success.

1. Pre-chop the veggies, meat, and any herbs and spices before starting to cook.
2. Assemble your oils and sauces before you start cooking so that they are all at hand.
3. Cut the ingredients so they require the same amount of cook time.
4. Cook the ingredients in separate batches or, if using a large pan, add the ingredients that tolerate longer cooking first, then push them out to the edge as you add new ingredients.

Stir-Fry Veggies (examples)
Bamboo shoots
Beans

Bell peppers

Bok choy

Broccoli

Carrots

Celery

Green onions

Green pea pods

Kohlrabi

Mushrooms, all kinds

Onions (yellow might work better than white or purple
   for stir-fry, but use what you have)

String beans

Water chestnuts

Stir-fry Proteins

Sirloin, tri-tip, ribeye, top loin (strip), tenderloin, shoulder center (ranch steak), shoulder top blade (flat iron), and shoulder petite tender. For beef, slice thin, and when possible slice against the grain. If the meat was frozen and is just thawing out, you can slice it more thinly as the firmness makes it easier to cut.

Chicken, cubed

Turkey, cubed

Shrimp, peeled and deveined

Scrambled egg

Tofu

If you have extra time, you can marinate your protein for one to twenty-four hours. Marinating keeps moisture in and also tenderizes the tougher cuts of meat, making just about any cut of beef and pork suitable for stir-fry.

To marinate, combine an acid (wine, sherry, vinegar) with a salty sauce (soy sauce, hoisin sauce, fish sauce, oyster sauce) and optional other ingredients (sugar, molasses, chopped garlic, chopped green onions, chopped ginger, chiles, five spice mix) and stir in the meat slices. Google or do a YouTube search for "marinade" with the ingredients you have on hand from each category to find full recipes. Always marinate in the fridge, covered. After you've removed the meat, discard the marinade, as cooking with it will impart off flavors and risks bacterial contamination from being infused with raw meat.

Zoodles

Instead of pasta, use fresh (not frozen, they're too mushy) zucchini noodles or butternut squash noodles. Zucchini noodles are just spiralized zucchini, and you can make them yourself with a spiralizer. Zoodles are good raw simply dressed with olive oil, salt, and parmesan, or mixed with fresh basil or tomatoes, or with a hot, meaty sauce like a Bolognese poured over them. You can also use the Upgraded Sauce recipe from Chapter 12 (Phase I: Metabolic Rehab: Baby Steps). The warm sauce heats the raw zoodles, and they retain enough texture to add a slight crunch.

You can find fresh zoodles at grocery stores like Target and Trader Joe's, and more stores are stocking them every day.

Nutrition in 1 medium zucchini, spiralized (about 1 cup zoodles), raw: 30 Calories; Carb, 6 g (Fiber, 2 g); Protein, 2 g; Fat, 1 g

Keto Casserole

Keto casseroles are one-dish wonders and get you veggies plus protein in a savory combo. They typically take about 20 minutes to prep and 30 minutes to cook enough to feed a family of six.

You can find keto casserole recipes on Google and YouTube. You can even search for specific ingredients by typing "'keto casserole' recipe using ground beef," or "'keto casserole' recipe using chicken and broccoli." There are currently almost a million results for "keto casserole recipe" right now and more popping up every minute, so there's a good chance you can find several your whole family will love.

Note: Making keto casserole as a side dish is a great way to convert veggie haters into veggie lovers, since it's hard to say no to broccoli that tastes like cheese and bacon.

Bare Naked Burger and Salad

Did you know that the original burger, from Hamburg, Germany, was bunless? Legend has it that at the 1904 World's Fair, the vendor selling hamburgers ran out of plates. Improvising, he bought some rolls from the vendor next door, sliced them in half, and voilà, the American burger! An instant hit. But don't be afraid to go back to basics; as long as you have access to a plate, knife, and fork, use them. You won't miss the bun for long.

You can use any kind of ground beef to make your burger, from full-fat (70%) to the lean extreme (95%). I try to use pasture-finished beef, which is often lean. This means when I make burgers, I add stuff to keep it moist. For each pound of ground beef I use an egg, a quarter of an onion, finely chopped, and 1 to 2 tablespoons wheat germ along with salt and garlic. Adding a few generous splashes of Worcestershire sauce to the raw meat makes for incredibly savory and delicious burgers.

After browning one side on medium heat in a saucepan for 5 to 10 minutes, flip, add as much cheese as humanly possible, cover, and cook on low for another 5 to 10 minutes or so till done and the cheese is melted. Burger enthusiasts can argue endlessly over whether you need to grill or cook uncovered or how thick it needs to be, but in my medical opinion there's no way to do it wrong other than overcooking.

If you come home tired and need to take the shortest line between the front door and a burger on your plate, try this trick. Buy your ground beef in one of those one-pound square packages. Open carefully and cut as many ½-inch slices as you want to make. Add to a hot pan with enough oil to coat, cook on medium for a few minutes till cooked about a quarter of the way through, flip and optionally sprinkle tops with Worcestershire, salt, and garlic powder before you add cheese. Cover and cook until desired doneness. If you're good, you don't ever touch the meat so you never have that typical burger-night battle to remove grease between your fingers. (Or you can buy pre-shaped patties, but those don't look right to me.)

Soup Is Good Food

Whether your favorite soupy stew is chili or chicken noodle, beef stew or Bolognese, pho or French onion, you can modify the recipe so that it's more nutritious by making one of the carb swap-outs from the chart on page 246 in Chapter 12.

For example, when rice is integral to the soup, swap it out for riced cauliflower, and chances are nobody but you and your rice cooker will notice.

When beans are a major player, cut the normal amount down by a third to a half and amp up the meat and/or the veggies. If it's potatoes you need to exchange, great northern beans or cannellini beans make a more nutritious edition. You can buy beans canned, but best to buy them dried and sprout them for a few days. The process of sprouting beans improves them in much the same way that sprouting wheat berries, discussed on page 198, improves sprouted grain breads.

If your soup requires noodles, use shredded cabbage. I kid you not—it works.

The keto/low-carb swap-out for the crusty bread atop French onion soup is to top generously with Gruyère and then brown in the broiler. There's always a solution, and if you can't come up with it on your own, consult with Chef Google.

Steamed Veggies

One of the most overlooked and healthiest ways to make fast, delicious veggies is to steam them, then drizzle over your favorite sauce. You can steam in the microwave, but because microwaves can break down plastic, I avoid extended microwaving and prefer steaming in a steamer on the stove top. If you don't have a steamer, the $30 investment will change your relationship with veggies forever. The technique applied to broccoli below works on any vegetable. The trick is to cut big chunks down into uniform sizes. Cutting increases the surface area and accelerates the steaming process, and uniformity prevents overdoing the skinny pieces.

Steamed Broccoli

Steam broccoli on the stovetop by bringing about an inch of water to a boil in a steamer. While water is heating, chop broccoli into even, bite-size pieces. Add broccoli to steamer and turn down heat so that the water is just boiling. Cover loosely so a little steam can escape, ideally using a glass top so you can see the color change that indicates doneness.

Test with a fork to ensure broccoli is cooked through. The fork should pass all the way through with just a little resistance. A soggy texture and tepid brown color means it's overdone and won't taste nearly as good.

Other easy-to-steam veggies: asparagus, Brussels sprouts, carrots, cauliflower, kale, string beans.

Garlic Butter

While your veggies are cooking, chop a couple cloves of garlic, or push through a garlic press. Once veggies are done, dump hot water from the pot, then add butter to the hot pan first, and then add garlic in the puddle of butter. Salt to taste and stir occasionally. If you need more heat, keep the butter on low until it starts to smell fragrant. Drizzle over your veggies when ready. The longer the garlic sits in hot butter, the milder the flavor—to a point. When overcooked, garlic can get quite bitter.

Drizzle Steamed or Pan-Fried Veggies with

- Fresh garlic butter, made per instructions above
- If you don't have fresh garlic, you can mimic Olive Garden's garlic butter spread: in a food processor, combine butter with garlic powder, onion powder, and parsley flakes
- Equal parts fish sauce and soy sauce
- Cheese sauce (Chef Sandra's All-Star recipe on page 305)

Low-Carb Veggies and Relative Steaming Time

Arugula and spinach: 3 minutes

Broccoli, cauliflower (florets—stems take longer unless sliced to ¼ inch thin), and green beans: 5 to 7 minutes

Asparagus: 5 to 10 minutes, depending on thickness

Brussels sprouts, carrots, and turnips: 10 to 20 minutes—slice in half to steam faster; for extra flavor, after steaming, give a thin coat of oil with salt and pepper and quick broil in the oven to get a little char

Edamame (shells removed): 15 minutes

Kale: 20 minutes

The Land of Salad

There's almost nothing easier than chopping things up and tossing them into a giant bowl to make salad.

A simple rule for making a delicious salad to accompany dinner is the Rule of 4s: Use 4 cups of veggies per person with at least 4 different colors, and get explosive flavor from 4 condiments or oils.

Step 1. Instead of mixing salad in a big bowl and serving in a dainty dish, serve in big bowls. You want that space because for your salad to be a flavor adventure, you need to be able to poke around with your fork and toss stuff out of the way to see what different combinations taste like.

Step 2. Add 4 cups of leafy greens like baby greens, spinach, kale, arugula, or romaine.

Step 3. Add 3 additional colorful veggies like carrots, purple onion slices, chopped celery, sprouts, frisée lettuce, red bell peppers, cucumbers, fennel, or radish.

Step 4. Add your choice(s) of the following toppings:

- Crumbled or shaved cheeses like Gorgonzola, feta, Parmesan, or Romano
- Nuts and seeds like pine nuts, roasted and salted pistachios, cashews, sprouted pumpkin seeds, or sprouted sunflower seeds
- Pickled or preserved vegetables like olives, roasted red pimento, hot chili peppers, pepperoncini, fresh or roasted garlic, artichoke hearts (the more pungent, the more you should mince finely to distribute)
- Roasted veggies like beets, garlic, artichoke hearts—all of which you can buy pre-roasted in higher-end grocery stores.
- Slow carb like chickpeas (a.k.a. garbanzo beans), heart of palm, water chestnuts, or roasted chestnuts
- Fresh or dried fruits like blueberries, dried cranberries, or apple or pear slices

Step 5. Dress it up. Get good-quality oils and vinegars and follow the per-serving rule of 2 tablespoons of oil per ½ to 1 teaspoon of vinegar.

- Mediterranean, all-purpose: cold-pressed olive oil with balsamic or apple cider vinegar. Optional herbs and spices: Italian seasoning, basil, garlic powder, onion powder. Add salt to taste, usually ⅛ to ¼ teaspoon.

- Asian, all-purpose: Unrefined peanut or sesame oil, apple cider or rice vinegar, Kikkoman soy sauce, Dijon mustard. No need for salt when you use soy sauce.

Let's take a moment to highlight the power of dressings to transform your salad. You can have the exact same veggies in your salad as you did yesterday, but simply getting a good-quality unrefined peanut oil (or roasted peanut oil) and a splash each of vinegar and soy sauce and—*bam!*—you're on the streets of Singapore enjoying a wholly new salad experience.

The land of salad is a kind of Eden where almost everyone plays nice together. So be daring and try new combinations.

What Else Can I Eat for Dinner?

Any dinner that is vegetable-oil-free and keeps your total daily net carbs—meaning you can subtract half the fiber—at 50 grams or less.

#GOALS

You're ready for Phase II when:

- You've continued to avoid snacks, base your breakfast, lunch, and dinner on the five rules, and found that you've not been hungry at all for three or four days.
- You have enough energy late morning and late afternoon that you don't get overly hungry or tired at meals.
- After a long busy day, you've had enough energy to prepare a healthy dinner.

You're not ready for Phase II if:

- You've experienced any of the eleven hypoglycemia symptoms in the past week. (This applies even if mealtime was later than normal—hypoglycemia is always a red flag.)

- You don't feel like you are ready to skip meals on occasion.
- You're in a hurry to get to Phase II so you can lose weight.

Remember, if you don't want to cut your carbs to follow a keto-style diet, you don't need to. You can stick with Baby Steps until you are ready for Phase II, and you will gauge whether or not you are ready by the same criteria above.

14

Phase II

Lasting Weight Loss

IN THIS CHAPTER YOU'LL LEARN TO

- Use intermittent fasting and other strategies to safely cut calories and accelerate weight loss.
- Reboot your appetite control system so it can "see" the body fat you have and use it to generate energy.
- Extract your sweet tooth and start craving real foods.

Now that your snacking habit is a distant memory, you've gone days without being hungry, and you have the energy to think through the process of making a meal so you're not tempted by tiredness to take the drive-through route home, you're finally ready to start burning some serious body fat.

Your past struggles with fatigue and hunger are over. You're ready and able to tackle the consequences of the struggles: excessive body fat. And you are ready to do that because the cause of those struggles was toxins in your body fat. That toxic body fat has already been significantly mitigated by the work you've done so far.

Your mitochondria (Fatburn System 1) are working better, so you have more energy all day. Your hormones (Fatburn System 2) are working better, so your body fat is ready to release its stored energy between meals. And you've been detoxifying your body fat (Fatburn System 3) of its unstable fatty acids so that when your cells receive body fat, they can generate more energy from it.

Here in Phase II is where the magic happens in the appetite centers of your brain (Fatburn System 4).

When you started Phase I, your body fat was visible to your eyes but invisible to your brain. You could see it, you knew it was there, but the body-composition center in your brain had no idea. Your brain was not letting you burn your body fat because it did not believe you had enough to spare. Now, after all the work you've done, your brain can finally start to see what your eyes have been seeing all along: that you have energy to burn.

This is the reason you've been less hungry.

Now that your brain can see your body fat, it can help you burn it by way of the sympathetic nervous system, sending electrical signals directly to your adrenal glands between meals. Your adrenal glands will now support your goal of weight loss by producing a fast-acting hormone called adrenaline, which travels through your bloodstream to activate your body fat. Once it arrives, it stimulates individual fat cells to get busy releasing fat. Adrenaline also ensures more blood flows through your body fat so the fatty acids released can rush out to energize the rest of your body.

The longer you go between meals, the more adrenaline your body produces and the more energized you get. That means it's important to go as long as possible between meals, which includes skipping meals. In other words, fasting. Another term for fasting recently popularized is "time-restricted feeding." In time-restricted feeding you only eat during a certain window of time during the day. Some people choose to set their window earlier than others. Some choose to set it to just a few hours per day. To get the max benefits of the time-restricted feeding strategy, you really do need to skip the equivalent of a meal. Most folks who "restrict" between normal eating hours of, say, 8 a.m. and 8 p.m. are not cutting very many calories and may not see much of a change.

The most wonderful thing about a healthy metabolism is that, even though you won't feel hungry, after you've gone a long time without eating, when you break your fast—whether you do this morning or night—your food will taste a whole lot better. In fact, the healthier the food, the more delicious and satisfying it will be.

PHASE II GOALS

Phase II is all about mindful eating. By fasting, you learn to get in touch with true hunger—the hunger for nutrition rather than for energy. You can free yourself from arbitrarily eating according to the clock, and instead eat according to other priorities, like eating when it's most convenient for you to make a healthy meal. This means you can be in control of when you eat.

Being in control of *when* you eat also helps you control *what* you eat. Many folks who have adopted this kind of lifestyle find that traveling is a great time to practice skipping meals, because in many cases there's just no good food available. Now, rather than being distressed by the lack of healthy options, you can use it as an opportunity to burn your body fat and feel good about not putting more toxic fat or addicting flours and sugars into your body.

As far as macros for this phase, feel free to continue whatever has made you feel best so far, be it the keto-style macros from the Accelerated Plan, or the more relaxed carb restriction of the Baby Steps portion of Phase I. I'd recommend enjoying a range of net carbs on different days; some days drop down to 20 grams, and some days eat up to 60 or 70. If you exercise for a couple hours, you can sometimes go even higher.

Keep in mind, however, that if you find yourself feeling hungry again and you're not losing weight, you may be falling back into old habits of eating too much carb and not enough clean-burning fat.

Your most important goal in this phase is to set yourself up for long-term success by resetting your appetite back to normal. Most of the folks I work with have come to me with damaged metabolisms that distort the hunger experience so that it's all about energy and fuel. By the time they're ready to graduate, their hunger experience is all about nutrition. That's where you need to be for weight loss—and for life.

Being hungry for nutrition rather than energy makes life simple. Your cravings align with your body's needs rather than conflict with them. And it means you can eat relatively simpler foods as well. You can even eat the same six or seven dinners over and over and they'll taste pretty great each time because you're fulfilling your nutritional needs. One of my former patients says he now "eats boring food and lives an interesting life." When you do get curious about new dishes and want to spread your culinary wings a little more, you'll have the energy for experimentation.

You don't need to fast for days to accomplish the goal of resetting your appetite. Just skipping a meal every few days is the way to start. The more often you skip meals, the more often you practice burning body fat. The more often you burn body fat, the faster you can produce ketones and the more ketones you produce. Those ketones will supply plenty of fuel for your brain, reducing or even completely eliminating its need for sugar. The faster your body makes ketones, the more energized you feel and the better you can concentrate and problem solve.

You know concentration and problem solving are essential skills at work—whether your job is to run a company or a household. We don't talk about it enough, but concentration and problem solving are also essential skills for weight loss. You need to be on your game to come home after a long day to a fridge full of food and be able to transform raw ingredients into a tasty meal in time for everyone to get to bed.

Now that you're ready for intermittent fasting, you're ready to take on that challenge. So let's get started by going into a little more detail about the options available to you.

METHODS OF FASTING

When first starting out, you definitely don't want to fast all day. As was true when you first started, the key is baby steps. Start out with a *fast* fast by just skipping a single meal.

Skip a Meal

The widely accepted practice of eating three square meals is a by-product of the industrial age, when the workday pushed other meals to earlier in the morning or later at night, so workers lobbied for a midday break. What little information we have on eating habits before the industrial era suggests that when work life was not defined by punching a time clock, most folks ate one or two times a day, typically whenever it made sense for their particular lifestyle or as dictated by local culture.

Which meal you decide to skip is entirely up to you. I recommend picking the meal that will make your life easier by skipping it. For me, the answer is lunch. I don't want to bother bringing it, then figuring out when and where I'll eat it. My digestive system has always rebelled against eating while working—eating makes me tired and want to lie down. So for me, skipping lunch gives me energy and prevents me from feeling uncomfortable during the afternoon.

Some folks are so busy in the morning that it makes more sense to hit delete on breakfast. A minority of folks choose to skip dinner, though usually they also enjoy a relatively large breakfast and relatively late lunch.

You may find that skipping meals comes naturally to you, in which case this phase will be a breeze. Be sure, however, that you don't pad the skipped meal with snacks—often some folks do without really noticing. The first time you skip a meal and go all the way to the next meal without snacking, it may feel difficult, but that will get easier the next time, and the next. If you skip lunch more often than you skip dinner, you may find the first time you skip dinner surprisingly hard. Whatever you practice, it will get easier the more often you practice.

Time-Restricted Feeding

Another strategy is to set up guardrails around what time of day you can and can't eat. In this case, people choose a window of time to eat and otherwise don't count their meals. So for example, they'll only eat between 11 a.m. and 6 p.m. This strategy does not specifically prohibit snacking, and some people end up eating more food more often than they realize during that time window. Still, if it seems easier for you, then give it a go.

HOW OFTEN TO FAST

Start with just once or twice a week. How often you fast depends on how you feel during that first experiment.

If you find you get really hungry after skipping a meal, so hungry that you're famished by the time you break your fast and feel drawn to overeat or eat foods you know are not so good for you, then maybe it's better to go back to Phase I for a few more weeks before trying again. This is actually quite common because folks get so excited about the prospect of losing weight that they'll begin Phase II before truly mastering the goals of Phase I, when they're still metabolically ill-prepared to cut calories. There's no harm done and no shame in going back for a little while before trying again. Chalk it up to learning a bit more about your metabolism.

If you pulled off the experiment in meal skipping without a hitch, then try it two or three days a week for a couple of weeks. You can dial it up or down at any time.

When you practice fasting in any form, it's especially important to get plenty of salt with your meals. Some folks notice they'll experience headaches or dizziness or brain fog and wonder what's going on. If you feel hungry when this happens, it could be hypoglycemia, which means you're not quite ready for fasting, and I recommend going back to Phase I for a little while—either the Baby Steps or the Accelerated Plan. If you don't feel hungry, it could simply be that you need more salt. This is very common, and sometimes you have to resort to taking ¼ or ½ teaspoon or so by spoon and chasing it down with a few ounces of water. It's also very important to supplement according to Rule #5, in Chapter 11, when you restrict calories, and you are (most likely) restricting calories on the days you're skipping meals.

If you feel tired during the tail end of the fasting interval, it's also possible that your fatigue is just lack of sleep. Try it again in a few days after you've slept better (see section on chronic sleep deprivation on page 312 of Chapter 15).

HOW LONG TO FAST

There's no clear benefit to fasting for days in a row unless it makes your life easier. I would definitely not try that until you've been in Phase II for several months. And even so, I would limit the duration to three days maximum. Remember, the point of fasting is cutting calories in the easiest possibly way. So if you've cut your calories by just skipping a single meal, then you're fasting for long enough to derive the benefits of Phase II.

Now that fasting is popular, some people are taking it too far. They're turning it into a competition, which takes the focus off how you're feeling and shifts it to comparing how you're doing against other people who may have nothing in common with you, metabolically or lifestyle-wise. Whatever you do, please don't start making fasting a competitive sport.

I've seen fasting gurus suggest that you can fast as long as you want and nothing bad will happen. That is too extreme a suggestion, in my opinion, particularly since we have very little research on the physiology of fasting. Much of what we do know comes from studying those who fasted as a form of protest and who were willing to die for their cause, and many did—in just a few weeks.

I've also heard it said that fasting spares muscle protein compared to other forms of calorie restriction. That may be true, but only up to a point. Multiple studies have shown that participants on a 1000-calorie-or-fewer meal plan do lose as much as a pound or two of muscle mass over the study periods, which is usually at least twelve weeks. We know from studying folks fasting for up to four days that there was little measurable muscle protein loss as far out as seventy-two hours, but there was a trend toward notably diminished muscle mass during the fourth and last day before the experiments stopped. There are no longer-term fasting studies I've found that show a muscle-sparing effect.

You might hear about folks doing broth fasts and fat fasts. While there's nothing wrong with that if it works for you, it's not accurate to call it a fast if you're consuming calories. It's calorie restriction, very much like a crash diet, but instead of consuming grapefruit or cabbage soup, you're consuming broth. So why not call it what it really is: a bone-broth crash diet? It may seem like a fussy point, but calling it a crash diet helps highlight the potential for nutritional deprivation over the long term.

There is also a lot of talk around fasting for cancer prevention and treatment invoking the term "autophagy." "Autophagy" refers to a form of cellular housekeeping where the parts of a cell that are old and worn out get disassembled and taken apart while the cell as a whole continues to thrive. The folks promoting autophagy suggest that you need to be in deep ketosis only achievable with fasting for three or more days or you are a setup for cancer and other chronic disease. That is not true.

Cellular housekeeping, including autophagy, occurs on an ongoing basis—at least when your metabolism is healthy. The inflammation that accompanies metabolic dysfunction interferes with this process, but you don't need to fast for days to repair your metabolic function and restore autophagy. Following this program does both.

INTRODUCING NEW FOODS

For any new way of eating to be sustainable, you have to enjoy what you eat. And one key to that is variety. Another is a sense of adventure. Introducing new foods solves both.

Whether you've never tried a food before, or you did and currently believe you don't like it, there is a simple trick that helps your body accept the new food and enjoy it: realizing that enjoying new and different foods is actually a learning process.

One of my patients in Napa was a retired preschool teacher who babysat for a few preschool-age kids on weekday afternoons. After we met, she bought herself a copy of *Deep Nutrition* and happily resumed eating foods she loved but had been avoiding because she thought they were bad for her high blood pressure and cholesterol—salted fresh tomato slices, dill pickles, cheese, pepperoni. She also realized that the cookies and brownies she was giving the kids were not doing them any good.

When she mentioned at one of our visits that she had also been feeding the children these healthy foods instead of the treats they'd grown to expect, I was very eager to learn how she pulled off that magic act. She said it was easy. All she did was wait until the kids came in from playing outside, at the time she usually gave them cookies, to announce she didn't have the cookies ready yet, so sorry, but they were welcome to share what she was eating. She made sure they knew that if they didn't like what she was eating, they didn't have to finish and that anyone who wanted could still get a cookie as soon as she was done with her food. Two of them were naturally curious and managed to charm the third by gently convincing him he didn't want to be the only one left out.

That's how we help our children with this learning process. And we can help ourselves as adults. You can apply this same kind, gentle encouragement to train your own taste buds to appreciate nutritious foods you've not tried before. Start with something someone you know has told you they like, maybe a new vegetable, a cheese you haven't tried, a nut or nut butter you've passed over before, and buy as little of it as you can. Then the first time you try it should be when you are a little bit hungry, and just try one bite. If you're not in love, then don't finish it. But do repeat the procedure again.

Child psychologists say kids need to try a new food ten times before their taste buds decide if they like it or not, so give your taste buds the same training period.

Common foods people select to retrain for are super healthy and readily available, like fermented pickles or kimchi, liver pâtés and canned fish (like bone-in sardines). Implement the craving-creation strategy of your choice (see above). Then eat 2 to 3 ounces of the retraining food. Repeat every few days or at least once weekly. Give it twelve weeks. If it fails after that time period, you can try again in a few months, but also you can just accept that you don't like that food—again, there's nothing wrong with that!

CREATING CRAVINGS FOR SPECIFIC FOODS

Another step you can take to expand your dietary repertoire is to teach your body to do more than just *accept* healthy food; you can teach your body to crave it. This is another key to lasting success, and it prevents you from ever feeling the least bit like you're living in a state of deprivation.

Let's talk about how exactly you are going to be able to stop craving junk once and for all and start craving real nutrition.

The key has to do with letting our *appetite* function as designed.

Back when I was growing up, before cell phones and electricity, snacks were for babies, or kids with moms who entertained a lot and fed leftover hors d'oeuvres to hungry neighborhood children. Working-class parents like mine had a knee-jerk phrase to quiet any predinner whining for food: "You'll ruin your appetite."

A wise mom I met a few years ago told me "hunger is a great teacher." That is definitely true. It's also easy to forget when hunger is associated with intolerable hypoglycemia symptoms.

There are two strategies for creating cravings for healthier foods.

The first is to plan your post-fast meal. On a day where you are going to fast at least 10 hours while awake, plan to introduce the food at that ten-plus-hour time point.

The second is to plan your post-exercise meal. If you are in the habit of exercising regularly, go work out on an empty stomach. After you've completed your workout, wait at least an additional hour before eating again. If you are not in the habit of regular exercise, you can try this after a workout, but be aware that until you develop a routine around exercise, you may find that you're too hungry to wait that extra hour.

A "MEAL PLAN" FOR FASTING

The last two chapters gave you meal plans and recipes to prepare your metabolism to burn fat. Now that you're ready to burn fat, it's time to start planning meals. A meal plan for fasting may sound like an oxymoron. But as you just read, the tandem goals of this chapter include (1) skipping meals to force your regenerating metabolism to burn fat and (2) finding new foods you enjoy and new dishes you look forward to eating.

As with the last two chapters, I'm not going to overload you with detailed recipes for dishes you may or may not even end up liking. Instead, I'm going to give you easy-to-read tables of ideas on how to take advantage of the many clean-burning fat recipes on the web. I'll also give you more detailed instructions for just a few essential recipes and introduce you to a few essential skills that will help you master the art of making fast, healthy meals.

Even if you eat just two meals a day, the first one is usually smaller than the second. The pattern many folks take as they make Phase II a lifestyle is to have a light morning or afternoon meal, maybe just coffee or tea with a small bite to eat, and a much larger meal in the evening. That much larger meal needs to provide most of the nutrition you'll need, so I call it a supermeal. Instead of giving you ideas for three meals in this chapter, I'll give you ideas for a small meal and a much bigger supermeal.

PHASE II FAST AND FLAVORFUL
ASTERISK INDICATES SUPERFOOD

IDEA	DESCRIPTION
Morning Coffee or Tea	coffee or tea with added half and half or coconut cream or blended with butter and collagen*
Finger Foods	1-2 oz your favorite cheese with 1-2 oz your favorite nuts
Fast Fish	1 can sardines* with anchovies or sauerkraut* 1 can smoked oysters with mustard
Broth Bowl	1-2 cups bone broth* microwaved 1 minute top with: nutritional yeast,* sprouted pumpkin seeds, optional dessicated liver* and/or bone marrow* powder
Wurst "Crackers" Ever*	liverwurst* or bratwurst* slices on cheese slices topped with horseradish mayo & mustard
Kimchi Eggs	hard boiled egg slices or eggs any style with kimchi* (or avocado)
Sashimi/Sushi	sushi is available at most grocery stores and airports; skip some or all of the rice

FAST AND FLAVORFUL SMALL MEAL IDEAS

These ideas are intentionally more "challenging" to the taste buds, not because I want you to force yourself to eat them if you don't like them, but because I have faith that if you try them when you are truly hungry, when your appetite has been whetted—after having gone a long time without eating—you will find that you actually enjoy some foods you never expected you could.

Morning Coffee or Tea

1 to 2 cups of coffee with enough cream, coconut milk, or half-and-half to taste delicious. You can also blend with butter and/or collagen/cartilage powder, the bone-broth mimic discussed in Chapter 11 (Five Rules That Fix Your Fatburn). As you learned, bone-broth mimics are one of the few supplements I recommend, but there's no point in buying them until you are in Phase II. While your metabolism is still fixated on sugar, it will likely just break those collagen/cartilage powders down to burn as fuel. Your

body is not going to benefit from these supplements and, worse, they may even deepen your insulin resistance. Now that you've reduced both your body's sugar addiction and its tendency toward signal-jamming inflammation, those collagen and cartilage powders can better support your skin, hair, gut, and joint health.

Finger Foods

If you keep your fridge stocked with two or three of your favorite cheeses and several varieties of nuts and/or seeds, you're never more than thirty seconds away from a filling meal. If you travel, these keep best in separate containers, meaning keep the dry nuts and seeds separate from the cheese. There's no reason you need to make breakfast or lunch more complicated than this.

Fast Fish

Canned fish may be the best-kept superfood secret. Canned tuna is loaded with healthy proteins and goes great with so many salad condiments it's easy to whip up a simple tuna salad if you have the right mayo on hand. Smoked oysters in tins are surprisingly delicious, like bacon and fish had a baby together, and taste wonderful simply dolloped with a nice Dijon mustard. Canned salmon is loaded with both healthy protein and fats. When you choose skin-on and bone-in, you're getting both collagen-health-supporting glycosaminoglycans and bone-health-supporting minerals. Everything tuna can do, canned salmon can do better—from salad to patties to simply tasting great with cottage cheese, a squirt of lemon, and salt. I recommend you always have some fast fish in your cupboard. Lastly, sardines. I pop open a can, plop the fish on a bed of fermented sauerkraut, and enjoy as a kind of fishy salty salad. Tastes even better with a few anchovies.

All of these also make fast and easy travel foods. As always, you need to read ingredients to avoid the three *C* and three *S* oils and choose products canned in olive oil or water.

If you're not a current fish fan, these might take some getting used to. However, ready-to-eat fish is a perfect example of a food you might want to take the time to train your taste buds to tolerate or even enjoy by following the protocol recommended above. If you're just not there yet but do like the idea of convenience, you can buy canned chicken or canned pulled pork instead.

Broth Bowl

The idea here is to start with a flavorful broth and add foods that just need to be warmed. These are a few of my personal favorites as well as some that go over well with the folks at work. More detailed broth bowl ideas can be found in the Recipe section of this chapter.

Faux Pho

One of the best takeout options is pho, a Vietnamese soup based on an aromatic broth. Pho made in the authentic fashion, with bone broth, not boullion, is available in just about every midsize or larger city I've been to. If you get your pho to go, you get a massive amount of broth (and a massive amount of noodles, which you can discard). I've used the leftover pho broth as inspiration to combine all kinds of odd bits and pieces badly needing use in my fridge. No matter how bizarre, the magic of stock means the results end up tasting delicious and new. Here are a couple, just to illustrate how you really can't go wrong when you start with a stock that was made right.

Sausage and Kale Ravioli

Now that your metabolism is recovered, you can include regular pasta, ravioli, rice, or potatoes as long as the portion sizes are modest. Here's an example of what I mean by modest.

Heat 2 cups of stock in microwave or stovetop, add 3 ounces precooked sausage, 1 ounce of dried kale chips (I recommend simple flavors, not nacho cheese, for example—and because the kale chips are dried, it's like they've been precooked, and you need only reconstitute for instant veggies), and 2 jumbo ready-to-eat ravioli stuffed with cheese and spinach; heat again to warm if necessary.

400 Calories; Carb, 30 g (Fiber, 5 g); Protein, 25 g; Fat, 18 g

Grass-Fed Hot Dog Soup

How weird is this? And it's still good! (Thank you, pho!)

Heat 2 cups broth, add 2 grass-fed hot dogs (nutrition based on Trader Joe's), sliced, and 1 ounce kale chips, and sprinkle over 2 ounces precooked quinoa (skip this to reduce total carbs by 10 g).
430 Calories; Carb, 22 g (Fiber, 6 g); Protein, 30 g; Fat, 29 g

Wurst "Crackers" Ever

Liverwurst and braunschweiger are both superfoods. You can spread on a slice of toasted sprouted grain bread, or any of the slow-digesting carb crackers described in Phase I, but my favorite is to use a thin sliver of cheddar cheese and dollop with mustard and the same blend of horseradish and avocado oil mayo recommended on page 195 of Chapter 11.

Kimchi Eggs

Kimchi is a live-culture fermented cabbage and one of the most popular condiments in Korean cuisine. It's readily available in most health food stores and increasingly common in grocery store chains. It's another of the foods that you might want to consider "training" your taste buds to enjoy. Regular consumption in cold and flu season is a great way to support your immune system and anecdotally has helped folks to avoid sickness when everyone around them is contagious.

Hard-boiled eggs taste great smashed into a bowl with kimchi.

Sashimi/Sushi

Raw fish is a superfood, as is all raw animal-based protein, because you get more bioavailable protein per gram from raw than you do after cooking. If you want to avoid rice, order sashimi instead of sushi.

PHASE II SAMPLE SUPERMEAL OPTIONS

IDEA	DESCRIPTION
The Land of Salad Leafy Edition	Per person: 4 cups of greens, 4 colors of veggies, 4-8 ounces protein, delicious dressing*
Giant Salad, Antipasto Edition	Mediterranean veggie preserves, beans, cooked chicken, sliced cured meats, olive oil, and herbs*
Good Soup	Per person: 2 cups of broth, 4-8 ounces precooked or fast-to-cook protein, 1-2 cup precooked or fast-to-cook veggies
Brined and Slow Cooked or Insta Pot	Brine a massive amount of chicken or pork, slow cook in the brine, accompany with high-fat salad like slaw
Roast Dinner	Oven roasted whole chicken with beans and Brussels sprouts, oven roasted lamb shoulder with carrots and turnips, roast beef with beets and green pepper
Exotic Meats	Liver, tripe, beef tendon, tongue, heart—these cheap cuts offer extreme nutrition. They're not for the faint of heart but something to aspire to.

The SUPERMEAL is designed for the days when you skip one or more meals. These are ideas to maximize your nutrition so that the food you eat will get you the most bang for your calorie buck. Now that your metabolism is healthier, calorie restriction on your meal-skip days facilitates both fatburn and weight loss. Asterisks indicate that there are sample recipes below in the Recipe section.

WHAT ELSE CAN I EAT IN PHASE II?

Phase II is your forever phase. Unlike Phase I, where we were trying to fix your metabolism using special nutritional hacks (slow-digesting carbs and keto macros in Baby Steps and the Accelerated Plan, respectively), here we are focused on curating a lasting relationship with healthy food.

The only limitations regarding ingredients are those you learned in Chapter 11 (Five Rules That Fix Your Fatburn). Stay away from vegetable oils, choose slow-digesting carbs rather than starchy foods or sweets, consume those slow-digesting carbs consciously—in moderation (60 to 70 grams or less per day)—and be sure to drink water and seek salt. Continue to avoid snacking, and be mindful about how often you have after-meal treats and desserts. On occasion, you can enjoy any sweetener you want, be it granulated sugar, maple syrup, honey, or what have you. These are to be treated as you would treat a spice—use to add an element of sweetness, not to overpower you with it. Same goes for your carbs, like flours, noodles, potatoes, pizza, and rice, which you can also consume on occasion instead of the healthier slow-digesting carbohydrate options. You can also use refined white flour if that's the best way to create a certain texture, but again it should be for that texture, not to fill you up with flour. For example, using a tablespoon of white flour to thicken a stock makes sense, or even to bake a cookie if you need it as a binder.

For this to be sustainable, you want to foster a sense of adventure. Anything under the sun that is vegetable-oil-free, gives you plenty of good fats, and does not taste overly sweet is fair game. Always remember that an essential part of fostering a healthy relationship with food is staying in control of what and how much you consume.

RECIPES

Broth Bowl

Superfood Soupy Side Dish with Sprouted Seed Croutons

This unusual soup boosts many B vitamins and minerals. Plus it boosts stuff you can't track, like branched chain fatty acids and glycosaminoglycans. It's weird but good. Don't say I didn't warn you.

Prep Time: 1 to 2 minutes, depending on microwave wattage
Serves: 1

   1–2 cups chicken bone broth (Pacific Foods and Kirkland both
      make good options)
   ½ ounce French Comté cheese, sliced

1 tablespoon nutritional yeast (Alive Foods is one of the few brands that does not spike its product with synthetic B vitamins)
1 ounce sprouted pumpkin seeds or sprouted sunflower seeds
Contents of 1 capsule each of desiccated liver, desiccated marrow fat, and desiccated trachea (optional)

Microwave broth until hot. Meanwhile, slice cheese into small pieces. Sprinkle cheese, yeast, and seeds over broth. If using the capsule contents, stir those in.

Gingery Poached Egg Soup

This simple, soothing soup is easy to pull together for a light lunch or dinner side, and please the tough crowd I work with. The eggs are poached in the broth and you can use whatever greens you have on hand. Recipe courtesy of Christen Rodgers.

Prep Time: 10 minutes
4 small or 2 big servings

1 tablespoon toasted sesame oil
5 thick (¼-inch) slices fresh ginger (or a teaspoon of powdered ginger)
2 cloves garlic, minced or sliced thin
6 cups chicken broth (homemade or boxed)
2 tablespoons non-MSG soy sauce or coconut aminos
12 ounces sliced or shredded cabbage
4 large cage-free eggs
Thinly sliced scallions

1. Heat sesame oil in wide pot over medium-high heat until shimmering. Add the ginger and garlic and cook, stirring constantly, until the garlic is just golden brown around the edges, about 1 minute.
2. Add the broth and soy sauce (or coconut aminos) and bring to a boil.
3. Add cabbage to the boiling soup, stir to combine, and bring back to a boil. Lower the heat to maintain a simmer and crack each raw egg into small ramekin/bowl, then carefully lower it into the soup (this will help

ensure the yolk doesn't break). Keep the eggs as far apart from each other as possible. Simmer undisturbed until the whites are set but the yolks are still runny, 3 to 4 minutes. Serve immediately, topped with scallions.

Leftovers can be stored in an airtight container in the refrigerator for up to 4 days.

Leafy (Side) Salads

Wilted Spinach Salad with Warm Bacon Dressing (plus bacon)

It's a shame to waste bacon grease, and the waste becomes pricey considering that thick-sliced bacon from humanely raised pigs can cost a dollar a strip. So at our house, we always save any extra bacon fat in easy-to-clean glass rame-kins in the refrigerator, where it stays good for weeks to months and can be used in place of butter to cook things like eggs, meat, and veggies. If you don't have any bacon fat in the refrigerator already, you can fry up 6 pieces of thick-sliced bacon to medium crispiness. Place bacon on a paper towel to drain. Since no human can resist eating bacon after frying it up, you might as well crumble a few strips over the finished salad.

Prep Time: 15 minutes   Total Time: 20 minutes
Serves: 2
253 Calories; Carb, 8 g (Fiber, 3 g); Protein, 7 g; Fat, 22 g

8 ounces (young) spinach
1½ tablespoons bacon fat
1 medium red onion
1 teaspoon red wine or apple cider vinegar (balsamic works too and adds some sweetness)
¼ teaspoon Dijon mustard

Remove any thick stems from the spinach. Wash and dry thoroughly and place into a large mixing bowl. Heat 1 tablespoon of the bacon fat in a frying pan at medium-low heat and add the sliced red onion. Cook down slowly for 10 minutes or so and allow it to caramelize and dry out a bit. Remove the onion and set aside. Add the remaining fat to the pan and whisk in the vinegar and Dijon mustard. Turn off the heat and allow the dressing to cool enough to safely taste and adjust seasoning. Gently fold the onion and the dressing into the spinach and serve immediately.

For additional protein, you can also serve the salad with sliced hard-boiled eggs. Thanks to the bacon-infused onion, even without bacon on top, this salad will still taste incredible, melting the cold hearts of salad haters everywhere.

Bacon-Infused Fennel & Red Onion Salad

This easy, delicious combination makes ordinary salad greens pop.

Serves: 1

    1 ounce finely chopped or grated fennel
    ½–1 ounce red onion sliced thin
    3–4 cups washed salad greens
    Olive or tea seed oil
    Apple cider vinegar
    1–2 finely chopped roasted pickled peppers

Brown the fennel and onion in bacon grease on really high heat for 1 minute. Put the salad greens in the bowl; then, while still hot, stir in some of the bacon-y fennel/red onion and oil/vinegar to wilt the greens a tiny bit. Top with the roasted pickled peppers. Add the rest of the dressing and stir. Avocado slices go great with this.

Full-Meal Super Salads

Antipasto

A super healthy, super easy meal, antipasto is a great opportunity to combine your favorite Mediterranean cheeses, meats, and condiments into one delicious bowl. You can dial the slow carbs up by adding beans and cutting out some or all of the meat.

Prep time: 30 minutes
Cook time: 0
Serves: 6
730 Calories; Carb, 14 g (Fiber, 5 g); Protein, 46 g; Fat, 55 g

Cut the following into bite-size pieces and combine in large bowl:

8 ounces cooked/roasted chicken meat

8 ounces sopressata

8 ounces Genoa salami

1 (14-ounce) can artichokes

2 large tomatoes

8 ounces sharp provolone cheese

8 ounces fresh mozzarella cheese

½ (12-ounce) jar roasted red peppers

Then add the following:

½ cup kalamata olives

¼ cup green olives

3 tablespoons red wine vinegar

¼ cup chopped, fresh basil

Sweet and Savory Salads

These single-serving salads include super simple dressings and require minimal chopping. Salads taste best with the freshest possible ingredients, so if you shop once weekly, make your salads early in the week. The addition of one or two premade gourmet and long-storing ingredients, like caramelized onion, or powerfully flavored simple additions like cranberry sauce or sautéed onion, makes salad creation (and eating) an endless source of mealtime variety and fun.

Cranberry, Shallot, Arugula, and Walnut Turkey

780 Calories; Carb, 19 g (Fiber, 3 g); Protein, 50 g; Fat, 57 g

2 tablespoons dried cranberries or cranberry sauce

1 tablespoon olive oil

2 cups arugula

4 ounces precooked oven-roasted turkey breast (Costco, or use nitrate-free deli-slices—I recommend Trader Joe's)

2 ounces crumbled gorgonzola cheese or goat cheese

2 tablespoons walnuts

¼ shallot sliced wafer thin

black pepper to taste

salt to taste

1 teaspoon apple cider vinegar

Option 1. Stir cranberry sauce together with olive oil before pouring over salad for flavor consistency. Note: Premade cranberry sauce in a jar keeps almost as long as jelly in the fridge.

Option 2. Convert to a mason jar lunch by layering the bottom with cranberries, shallots, cheese crumbles, and turkey, adding the oil and vinegar (and cranberry sauce if not using dried cranberries), then well-dried arugula, and lastly walnuts.

Mango, Avocado, Baby Spinach, and Hazelnut Chicken

720 Calories; Carb, 28 g (Fiber, 12 g); Protein, 52 g; Fat, 50 g

2 teaspoons mango chutney (Trader Joe's has a mango-ginger that works)

1 tablespoon olive oil

2 cups spinach

4 ounces precooked chicken (Wegmans, Trader Joe's)

1 ounce alfalfa or other sprouts

2 rings red onion sliced thinly

½ avocado sliced

1 teaspoon lemon juice or vinegar

1 ounce roasted hazelnuts

1. Stir mango chutney together with olive oil before pouring over salad for flavor consistency. Mango chutney in a jar keeps as long as jelly in the fridge.

2. Convert to mason jar lunch in a manner similar to Cranberry, Shallot, Arugula, and Walnut Turkey above.

Converting a Low-Carb Salad to a Slow Carb Salad

You can convert any low-carb salad into a slow carb salad by adding 15 to 30 grams of a slow carb. If you want to keep the calories low, then you can also pull back on the fat calories by reducing cheese, nuts, or oil by half.

Slow Carb Salad Toppings
Sprouted quinoa (sprout your own or buy ready-to-eat)
Sprouted grain bread croutons
Crumbled cracker croutons
Roasted beets (roast your own or buy ready-to-eat)
Artichoke hearts
Garbanzo beans
Water chestnuts
Hearts of palm
Bamboo shoots

Main Dishes

Chef Debbie Lee's Tangy Pork Butt

Chef Debbie Lee of MindBodyFork.com loves marinades that quickly convert into super easy meals, soups, and sauces. This marinade recipe hits the salty, savory, sweet, and sour flavors, making this surprisingly simple recipe delicious and fast.

To make marinade, for every pound of pork you will need:
4 bay leaves
4 garlic cloves
¼ cup tamari or soy sauce
½ cup apple cider vinegar
6–8 black whole peppercorns

Small thumb-size piece of ginger root, skin removed

1 tablespoon avocado oil to sear pork in Instant Pot

1 cup chicken broth/stock

1. Combine the bay leaves, garlic, tamari, vinegar, peppercorns, and ginger in a large enough bowl to accommodate pork and liquid. Marinate pork butt for at least 2 hours if not overnight.
2. Remove pork butt from marinade. DO NOT THROW OUT MARINADE. Strain liquid and set aside.
3. Put Instant Pot on Sauté mode. Once it reads hot, add oil and sear pork butt on all sides until browned. Add back marinade and broth. Cover with lid and set on high pressure; cook for 2 hours.

Enjoy it with some cauliflower rice or some black bean noodles!!!

Thomas Keller's Roasted Chicken Dinner

Thomas Keller is a magician in the kitchen. Unlike most magicians, he's more than happy to let you in on the tricks they use to keep seats filled at his Michelin-starred restaurants. This simple chicken is, apparently, something people wait months for. Just season it inside and out with salt and pepper, truss it as best you can with some butcher's twine, and roast it in the oven at 425°F. Let it rest (personally, I like resting birds upside down to allow the juices to percolate down into the breast) for about 20 minutes before serving.

You can turn the roasted chicken into a full meal simply by adding a few cups of veggies to the roasting pan—green beans, Brussels sprouts (halved), whole tomatoes, quartered onions or celery stalks. The recipe below includes a nice vegetable medley we often use. If you have the time, you might want to steam the Brussels sprouts for 3 minutes before roasting them, but it's not necessary. Just coat the veggies with a thin coat of olive oil and salt and pepper and they'll be a perfect accompaniment to the roasted chicken. You can brine the chicken for a day or two in salt water, but Thomas Keller says you don't have to. And his is the final word.

Prep time: 10 minutes
Total time: 1 hour

Serves: 4

700 Calories; Carb, 24 g (Fiber, 9 g); Protein, 49 g; Fat, 45 g

1 whole chicken, rinsed and patted dry
Seasoning (salt and pepper)
1 whole onion, roughly chopped
4 carrots
4 stalks of celery
1 pound of Brussels sprouts
½ pound of green beans
3 tablespoons olive oil

1. Remove chicken from refrigerator a full hour before you plan to roast it to bring it to room temperature.
2. Rinse and pat dry the chicken. Remove the wishbone if you'd like, as it makes carving easier.
2. Season it with salt and pepper, inside and out.
3. Truss the chicken with butcher's twine. Don't feel bad if this is frustrating. There are many techniques you can use.
4. Lightly coat the onion, carrots, celery, halved Brussels sprouts, and green beans in olive oil. Lightly season with salt and pepper and toss.
5. Preheat oven to 425°F.
6. Place chicken, breast side up, on a middle or high-middle oven rack in a roasting pan or cast-iron skillet on a bed of the celery and carrots.
7. Toss the onions into the pan.
8. Roast the chicken at 425°F. for an hour. A poke into the thickest part of the thigh should run clear. Food safety experts want the thermometer to read 165°F.
9. If the skin didn't brown, try broiling the chicken, on a high rack, for 5 minutes. You can, if you wish, drizzle a little balsamic vinegar over the veggies at this time, for a little acid.
10. Remove the chicken from the oven and let it rest, turned breast side down, for at least 20 minutes. Carve and serve.

Grilled Steaks with Peppery Lemon-Herb Marinade

You may already know this, but I'll mention it anyway: you don't want to cook steak—or hamburger, or chicken, or turkey, or eggs—straight out of the fridge. You want to temper them first, letting them get close to room temperature before you cook them. This allows for more even cooking and is particularly important for grass-finished cuts, which have less marbling within the meat (marbled meats are easy to cook and can be delicious, but indicate the animal suffered from a metabolic disorder induced by too much grain and too little activity).

Prep Time: 5 minutes
Total Time: 10 minutes

4 1½-inch-thick sirloin or rib eye steaks, preferably grass-fed
½ cup fresh lemon juice, plus 3 tablespoons
2 tablespoons olive oil
2 tablespoons minced fresh rosemary
2 tablespoons minced fresh thyme
6 teaspoons whole black peppercorns
1 tablespoon lemon zest
Salt to taste
2 cups mesquite or hickory-wood chips, soaked in water for at least an hour (optional)

1. Place the steaks in a nonreactive dish and pour ½ cup lemon juice over them.
2. In a food processor, combine the remaining lemon juice, olive oil, rosemary, thyme, peppercorns, lemon zest, and ¾ teaspoon salt and process into a paste.
3. Marinate the steaks in this paste, covered, for a couple of hours, or overnight, in the refrigerator.
4. If you're grilling, distribute the wood chips and fire up the grill until the chips start producing smoke.
5. Baste the steaks once or twice while they're cooking, and turn them when they're halfway through (8 minutes total for rare, 10 or so for medium rare).

6. Let rest for 10 minutes, then slice on the bias and season with a pinch of large-grain salt.

Seared Salmon with Mustard-Caper Sauce

This dish is so ridiculously easy, and it creates a quick, simple answer to dinner in just minutes. The trick to a delicious, crispy salmon skin is to pat the fish dry and season the skin side with only sea salt, then start cooking skin side down in a lot of oil. The salt absorbs moisture and helps crisp the skin.

Prep time: 10 minutes
Total time: 20 minutes
Serves: 4
640 Calories; Carb, 2 g (Fiber, 1 g); Protein, 47 g; Fat, 48 g

2 pounds salmon fillets, with the skin on
Salt and pepper
½ tablespoon olive oil, plus ¼ to ½ cup to sauté the salmon
2 tablespoons unsalted butter
1 tablespoon rinsed capers
Zest of ¼ lemon
1 teaspoon Dijon or brown mustard
2 tablespoons heavy cream
2 teaspoons coarsely chopped fresh dill
Garnish: 2 lemon wedges, 4 sprigs dill

1. Heat a heavy frying pan (cast iron works great) at medium heat.
2. Pat the salmon fillets dry and sprinkle a liberal amount of quality salt on the skin. That will serve as plenty of salt for the whole fish.
3. Grind a little white or black pepper onto the skinless sides of the fillets.
4. Add enough olive oil to liberally coat the bottom of the pan and heat until oil is hot enough to boil water (test by flicking water from your wet hand and listen for the sizzle).
5. When hot, place the fillets, skin side down, into the pan. As the salmon cooks, add ½ tablespoon oil, butter, capers, lemon zest, mustard, and heavy cream to a second pot. Bring to a simmer and stir often. Cook

salmon until color change shows that half the salmon is cooked through, then flip and cook for an additional minute or so.

6. Plate the cooked fillets. Add the chopped dill to the sauce and then taste for seasoning and adjust (remember, the salted side of the fillet has plenty of salt, so don't overdo it with the salt in the sauce). Sauce the fish. Garnish with lemon wedges and dill sprigs and serve.

Sauces and Dressings

Dijon Tamari

From Chef Debbie Lee of MindBodyFork.com

3 tablespoons Dijon mustard
½ cup rice vinegar
2 tablespoons tamari or soy sauce
Salt and pepper to taste
½ cup sesame oil

Whisk well. If you want to sweeten it, you can add a pinch of whatever sugar-free sweetener you like.

Sesame Miso

From Chef Debbie Lee of MindBodyFork.com

Yield: ½ cup

2 tablespoons miso (1 teaspoon for single serving)
2 tablespoons mayo (1 teaspoon for single serving)
½ cup rice vinegar or white vinegar or apple cider vinegar
    (1 tablespoon for single serving)
1 tablespoon tamari or soy sauce (½ teaspoon for single serving)
Salt and pepper
¼–½ cup sesame oil (1 tablespoon for single serving)

Whisk all ingredients together except sesame oil until emulsified, then add the sesame oil and whisk together. Keeps 2 weeks in the fridge.

Dijon Balsamic Vinaigrette

From Chef Debbie Lee of MindBodyFork.com

Single serving. Just stir in the bottom of your salad bowl, then add greens.

    2 tablespoons olive oil
    1 teaspoon Dijon mustard
    1 teaspoon balsamic vinegar
    ½ teaspoon honey (optional)
    Plenty of salt (½ teaspoon minimum)
    Pepper to taste

Sandra's All-Star Cheese Sauce

Courtesy of the LA Lakers' chef, Sandra Padilla, this cheese sauce has converted broccoli-haters into broccoli-eaters.

Serves: 6
280 Calories; Carb, 3 g (Fiber, 0 g); Protein, 9 g; Fat, 26 g

    1 cup heavy cream
    1 bay leaf
    4 ounces American cheese
    4 ounces cheddar (shredded)
    Salt and pepper to taste

Add ½ cup of cream, bay leaf, and cheeses to a medium saucepan. Add salt and pepper to taste. Cook over medium-low heat, stirring often until smooth and bubbly. Stir in remaining cream. Remove the bay leaf and serve. You can add 1 tablespoon tabasco or other hot sauce to give it some depth and heat.

Heavenly Cauliflower Mac and Cheese
(and Slow Carb Variations)

The key here is the cheese sauce. More gourmet than the simple cheese sauce above, this is made from a roux. When oven-baked till golden crispy and just browned along the edges in a casserole, this cheese sauce will bring you close to heaven pretty much no matter what you stick in it. You can even turn the recipe below into tuna casserole by adding mayo after the cheese is all melted in, along with numerous chopped veggies (diced celery and pimentos are delicious) and a few cans of tuna. Note: Other roux-based cheese sauce recipes do not require so much stirring but do require quite a bit more flour.

Yes, this takes longer than boxed mac and cheese. If you are having a mac and cheese emergency, you can cut the recipe in half, buy riced cauliflower and pre-shredded cheese, steam the cauliflower while making the roux, and simply pour the sauce over the steamed cauliflower. This will cut the time to about 20 minutes, or 10 for Olympic-level roux-based cheese-sauce makers. Or you could use Sandra's cheese sauce, above.

Prep time: 30 minutes
Total time: 55 minutes
Serves: 4
760 Calories: Carb, 14 g (Fiber, 2 g); Protein, 43 g; Fat, 60 g

   1 large head cauliflower, chopped into florets
   2 tablespoons butter
   2 tablespoons flour
   2 cups whole milk, warmed to room temperature
   2 pounds shredded sharp cheddar
   1/4 teaspoon finely ground black pepper
   1/4 teaspoon salt
   1/4 teaspoon garlic powder (optional)
   1/4 cup grated parmesan

   1. Heat oven to 275°F.
   2. Add cauliflower to an 8x14-inch casserole or equivalent, and place in the oven. Set timer for 15 minutes and remove when done. Turn oven temp up to 375°F.

3. Add butter to a medium-hot 2-quart saucepan, and when it starts to melt, add flour (white or spelt works better than wheat). Using a whisk, stir quickly to work the two ingredients together. You should see bubbles forming as the roux develops; stir constantly until the color just begins to darken and you notice a wonderful nutty aroma. Stirring constantly and slowly to blend, add about ¼ cup milk, keeping heat on high enough to generate a light but constant simmer, not a roiling boil. After a few minutes of stirring, it will thicken; add another ¼ cup. Repeat until all milk is added. Reduce heat to medium and stir another minute to thicken just a bit, then start adding cheddar cheese one handful at a time, making sure the last handful is melted before adding the next. Add black pepper, salt, and garlic powder, and stir until dispersed.

4. Remove partly dehydrated cauliflower from the oven, pour cheese sauce over, and stir to distribute evenly. Sprinkle top with parmesan. Bake for 20 to 25 more minutes or until top is golden brown and just crisping on the edges.

5. You can also substitute any of the lower-carb "noodles" mentioned in the Starchy Carb to Slow Carb swap-out chart on page 246 for the cauliflower. Particularly delightful is baked butternut squash.

Dessert

Luke's Lowest-Carb Keto-Compatible Crepe

Most crepe recipes call for equal amounts flour and eggs, by weight. This one makes three to four thin crepes and calls for just a tablespoon of flour per egg. Each tablespoon of flour has just 6 grams of carb, and you can probably make it work with ¾ tablespoon per egg once you get the hang of it.

1 egg
1½ teaspoons flour
1 tablespoon milk
Pinch of salt
1 tablespoon butter

Mix all ingredients except butter until smooth. In a hot pan, melt a teaspoon or so of the butter and pour a third or a fourth of the batter onto the side of the pan (as opposed to the middle). Tilt the pan around so that the batter coats as much of the pan as possible, for a nice thin crepe. In less than 30 seconds, the crepe will have formed up and bubbled up away from the pan. Flip the crepe and cook for another 10 seconds; then, with a spatula, remove it to a plate. Add a little more butter and pour in enough batter to make another crepe. After the batter's used up, melt a little additional butter in the pan and pour it over the crepes. For a savory crepe, you can roll sautéed minced shallots, sautéed mushrooms, lump crabmeat, or steamed spinach with the excess moisture squeezed out.

15

Troubleshooting and Frequently Asked Questions

IN THIS CHAPTER YOU'LL LEARN

- Eight places progress-blocking calories commonly hide
- How to combat frequently encountered complications of diet change
- How to find fatburning friends at work and at home

Even the best-laid plans run into hitches. So it's not at all uncommon for folks to need a little troubleshooting. This chapter covers some of the common problems my patients have experienced, and some of the solutions that have worked well for them.

PROBLEM: NOT LOSING WEIGHT

Eight Places Calories Hide

I've had the opportunity to troubleshoot with hundreds of my own patients, and to review cases with other physicians who specialize in weight loss. Time and again, if a patient isn't losing weight, the issue is that they eat more than they realize. If you are not losing weight in Phase II, any online calorie calculator will help gauge your baseline calorie needs, and if you're exercising they can also help you track your calorie burn. The website/app I recommend for tracking your food is Cronometer.com.

Below are the eight sources of excess or hidden calories, and reasons they creep up on you.

Your Meals, If You Are Not Measuring Accurately

Many people don't measure accurately, and will just "eyeball" how much oil they're using on their salads or in the pan or use silverware instead of measuring spoons (some silverware sets have "teaspoons" that actually hold nearly a tablespoon). Eyeballing is fine, after you've *trained* your eyeballs by actually using measuring tools. This is particularly crucial when it comes to fats and oils, because being off by half a tablespoon in three meals seven days a week can add up to over a thousand calories each week. Like every skill, accurate visual measurement requires disciplined self-education, period, so don't cheat yourself. Go ahead and double-check your work.

Overlooked Ingredients Not Added to Your Daily Totals

One of my patients was making a low-carb pudding recipe for breakfast and adding an optional nut butter but using the calorie count for the basic recipe without tallying the nearly 300 calories of nut butter she was adding. Another a patient of mine forgot to include the cooking fat she added to her skillet for breakfasts and dinners, which totaled 800 calories per week. Make sure to tally every single ingredient, no matter whether it seems significant or not. And make sure to input the ingredients you actually use; one patient underestimated her daily calories by 400 each day because, when building a dessert recipe in her app, she input coconut milk instead of the much higher-calorie coconut oil she actually used.

Small Pieces of Food Eaten Out of a Big Bag

Many folks eat foods like nuts and other snackables out of a big bag, a handful at a time. A handful of almonds has about 150 calories, a handful of macadamias almost 200. Most people can't stop at a single handful. If you have to eat on the go, then whether you eat in the car or from your purse, portion out your servings into smaller bags.

Calorie Bombs: Condiments, Desserts, and Smoothies

Coconut oil, chocolate, butter, nuts, and avocado are nearly ubiquitous in low-carb desserts and smoothies because they are loaded with healthy natural fats and some have other nutrients as well. But even though they are natural and healthy, they are still calorie bombs. The same goes for mayo.

Empty-Carb Calories

Foods like honey, dates, other dried fruits, agave nectar, and other popular natural sweeteners have as many calories as table sugar and high-fructose corn syrup. They do have a tiny bit of nutrition, but it's nominal and doesn't nutritionally justify making a meal out of anything sweet, or eating sweet things multiple times a day.

Empty-Fat Calories

Empty calories from fat are as much of a problem as empty calories from sugar. A few of the clean-burning fats I recommend for energy have relatively little nutrition, most notably macadamia nuts, ghee, MCT oil, and coconut oil. The other healthy fats, particularly butter, cream, and unrefined nut and seed oils, are more nutritious.

Reduced Activity

If you reduce your exercise level for whatever reason, or if you took a job that involved less activity, then you need to reduce your calorie intake accordingly.

This highlights another pitfall of relying on exercise to lose weight. Injuries are common even among professional athletes who have a team of people they work with to prevent injuries. If you're not a professional and you're training like you are, you're almost guaranteed to get hurt. Nearly every last one of my patients who jumps into an aggressive exercise program on their own ends up getting hurt. If they started their new diet at the same time they started exercising, they've often gotten used to certain portion sizes. While those portions may have promoted weight loss while burning an additional 200 to 500 calories or more, when the exercise stops, you need to adjust your intake accordingly.

Reduced Caloric Requirement

When you weigh more, your calorie requirements are higher than they will be after you lose weight. Not because your metabolism slows down, but because your body is doing less work just keeping you alive. You burn fewer calories doing the same activity because you're lifting less weight. You have fewer blood vessels and often your blood pressure drops as you get healthier, which means your heart has less work to do. When you eat less, your digestive system has less work to do. For all these reasons, when you lose any significant amount of weight, like 10 pounds or more, you need to eat fewer calories than before you lost weight or eventually you'll just gain the weight right back.

Let me give you an example. Let's say you're a fifty-year-old female weighing 180 pounds and you do light exercise a few days a week but your job is sedentary. To maintain your weight at 180 without gaining any more, you need 2310 calories per day. Now let's say you've lost 30 pounds and dropped down to 150. At the new, lower weight you only need 2090 calories each day. You have to continue to eat fewer and fewer calories the closer you get to your goal. This is difficult to achieve if you are tired and hungry all the time, which highlights the reason it's so important to get to the point you're burning body fat and producing ketones—because they give you that desire to move.

How Lack of Sleep Stalls Fatburn

It's very important to consider whether you're getting enough sleep. If you are chronically sleep-deprived, you may want to start making sleep more of a priority.

Chronic sleep deprivation sneaks up on us. Shawn Stevenson, host of the highly entertaining *The Model Health Show* and author of *Sleep Smarter*, points out that "nobody congratulates you for being a 'good sleeper.'" That's very true. In fact, many people consider sleep not a necessity but an indulgence, even a vice.

You may not have gotten decent sleep on a regular basis since college, or middle school. Many people are surviving on just five or six hours a night, when their body really needs seven or eight.

Some people need even more than eight. It's not that they're lazy. It's probably because they have to fight off numerous viruses, and we do that most effectively at night.

Some of us have been unlucky enough to contract viruses that don't leave our bodies. Chicken pox is one, which recurs as shingles. Mononucleosis, cytomegalovirus, parvovirus, and herpesviruses I and II are all examples of common viruses that keep our immune system busy at night.

If you've been following the plan, your hunger is well controlled, you're not snacking, you're not gaining weight (because that also can make us tired), but you've been struggling with low energy, sleep may be the missing piece. The first step to getting more sleep is setting a consistent bedtime and sticking to it. That means managing your time so you can start getting your head on the pillow with lights out and phone turned off earlier than you are now.

BINGE EATING AND SECRET EATING

Another reason for failing to lose weight is binge eating. Binge eating, unlike ordinary overeating, involves feelings of shame, loss of control, and need for secrecy. Somewhere between 20 and 50 percent of adults considering surgical treatments for obesity meet criteria for binge-eating disorder, but outside this select group binge eating is much less common, around 2 or 3 percent. While getting your metabolism into better shape is likely to be essential to making a full recovery, recognizing that you may be facing this complex issue, and getting help from an experienced professional, is likely to be beneficial as well.

PROBLEM: FEELING HUNGRY

Hunger is only harmful if you experience hypoglycemia symptoms that don't go away unless you eat. If you do have any of the eleven hypoglycemia symptoms associated with your hunger, then chances are you needed to add a little more slow carb to the meal you just ate, up to 30 grams or so, or a little more clean-burning fat, up to a tablespoon or so.

If you've already added the slow carbs and/or clean-burning fat as described above but still experience hypoglycemia symptoms with hunger, or if you experience those symptoms when you are not hungry, those symptoms may be due to another medical issue, some potentially serious and not related to diet, which should be evaluated by your doctor.

If hypoglycemia symptoms are not present, hunger may be associated with habit. This hunger is not long-lasting. It's driven in part by your stomach's hunger alarm clock, and shows up around the time you would normally have a snack or a treat or start thinking about your next meal. It's simply the empty-stomach-detecting hormone ghrelin signaling your brain to prepare the digestive system to accept food. You can turn this alarm clock off by retraining your brain so that it ignores ghrelin, and eventually ghrelin will stop pestering your brain. As long as you stay busy, this hunger should pass in a few minutes.

Tricks for Retraining Your Stomach Hunger Alarm Clark

If you're not doing something to distract yourself from your hunger, then you might need a little help ignoring ghrelin's pestering alarm. The good news is, these kinds of hunger signals and cravings usually disappear in five minutes or less. Here are a few tricks you can try to turn down the volume on the signal.

1. Drink a glass of water.
2. Chew sugarless gum.
3. Stand up and stretch or take a short walk outside.
4. Try to avoid locations where you might be exposed to the aromas of delicious foods.
5. Find a short task to complete and get busy with it.
6. Call someone you know for a quick friendly chat.

What Not to Do When Your Stomach Alarm Clock Is Ringing

1. Head to the kitchen at home.
2. Head to the break room at work.

3. Talk with a coworker about what you're doing for lunch.

4. Have a "healthy" snack or beverage—this just reinforces the habit.

Nausea Associated with Hunger

If your empty stomach makes you feel nauseated, it's a sure bet you will benefit from getting more gut-healing foods with your regular meals. If you absolutely need something to snack on to alleviate your hunger-induced nausea, make sure to get something salty and try to keep it under 25 calories. A few ideas for gut-healing, salty snacks to consider:

1. A dill pickle.

2. Half a cup of warm chicken stock or other bone broth.

3. Three or four pork rind crisps.

4. A quarter cup of kvass. Kvass is a fermented Slavic beverage made from beets or other foods. Zukay is my favorite brand.

PROBLEM: HEADACHE OR MUSCLE CRAMPS

Both these symptoms result from the fact that our foods are lower in minerals than they used to be due to soil depletion, so we have to take greater pains to get those minerals. The minerals that will help you avoid these symptoms are calcium, magnesium, zinc, and table salt (sodium chloride). To get them in adequate amounts, be sure to add salt to your meals, and supplement with the recommended minerals. If you don't add salt or eat salted preserved foods like cheese, pickles, and deli meats, or salted nuts and seeds, then you are getting almost no salt in your diet. Adding salt to your salads and vegetables makes them much tastier.

Minerals to Prevent Headaches and Muscle Cramps

- Magnesium oxide, 200–400 milligrams daily
- Zinc gluconate or picolinate, 15 milligrams daily
- Calcium citrate, 500 milligrams or 3 servings of dairy daily (see page 325, "What should I eat for bone health?")

- Potassium chloride, 99 milligrams, 2 or 3 per day
- Table salt, 1⅓–2⅔ teaspoons daily

The reason you need to seek out salt when you're on a lower-carb diet and avoiding processed foods is that you're reducing your intake of sodium at the same time as your insulin level is going down, and insulin helps your kidneys hang on to salt as well as other minerals. I take these minerals daily myself due to the soil depletion and almost always add salt to my veggies and dinner dishes.

If you are prone to migraines and notice headaches at any point in this diet, but find yourself caught without a snack, just find some salt, the kind you get from any cafeteria and most workplace break rooms. All you need is a pinch or two—pour it in a teaspoon or a cup and get it in you. If low salt is the cause of your headache, it can start helping within minutes. I've done this myself a few times, and got total relief of a pounding migraine.

PROBLEM: CONSTIPATION

Any drastic diet change can disrupt the gut flora in ways that lead to constipation. Over time you will develop new flora that help you digest your new diet, but it can take a few months.

Meanwhile, there are plenty of things you can do. If you used to eat a lot of whole grains and now you're eating a lot less, one of the best fixes for this is to add some fiber back in the form of flax meal, or just buy Metamucil or Citrucel and follow the instructions. Both Metamucil and Citrucel are available in a sugar-free formulation, which I recommend over the formulation with sugar. Docusate sodium, an over-the-counter non-stimulant laxative stool softener sold in capsules, also works well in this situation.

If you never ate a lot of whole grains, or if fiber and Colace do not work for you, try milk of magnesia. Another fiber-alternative is magnesium citrate, and the brand most of my patients use with success is Natural Vitality Calm Original (Unflavored), available online. Also, be sure to drink plenty of water daily and try to get lots of fresh veggies.

Avoid stimulant laxatives like Dulcolax and Ex-lax, which stop working after a few weeks.

PROBLEM: DIARRHEA

Loose stools and diarrhea not accompanied by heartburn are usually a result of adding too much new food at once (though it's also possible that your change in diet unmasked a side effect of a medication that you take). Your gut flora cannot digest absolutely everything. And when you change your diet, you actually change the kinds of species that live in your gut. As with constipation above, if you were eating a lot of whole grains, for example, and now are hardly eating any, then the billions of organisms that depended on your intake of grains are dying off, and during that process you may experience diarrhea.

The solution? Take a few steps back and then reintroduce the new foods after a week or so. If you had been following a low-fat diet, you might want to try going back to that for one or two of your daily meals, but not entirely if you can avoid it. Or, if you are eating a lot more veggies or nuts than usual, cut down your intake by half. Nuts can be another trigger, as can dairy (typically milk and cream but not usually yogurt or cheese).

While you add in some of the foods from your previous diet, you absolutely need to continue to avoid processed vegetable oils as much as you can, with a lower-priority focus on avoiding some or all of the processed carbs we've discussed.

PROBLEM: LACTOSE INTOLERANCE

Lactose is the most prevalent sugar in milk. Fermenting milk to make yogurt or cheese reduces the lactose, because the fermenting microbes digest it. Symptoms of lactose intolerance include bloating and diarrhea, usually starting within a few minutes of consuming lactose-rich dairy. Not all dairy has significant amounts of lactose, and everyone is sensitive to different amounts. This section will teach you about the kinds of dairy you might be able to consume even if you have lactose intolerance, and which kinds of dairy you will most likely need to avoid.

Lactose intolerance is not an allergy; it's caused by loss of the enzyme for digesting lactose, which leads to symptoms for unclear reasons—possibly a microbiome imbalance or drawing too much fluid into the gut, or both.

The symptoms are temporary and are not thought to cause anything more serious, like inflammatory bowel disease or celiac, although people with these conditions can be lactose-intolerant as a complication of their illness. You can buy lactase enzyme over the counter, which will temporarily replace your missing enzyme. If you get a good-quality supplement with lots of active enzyme, you may be able to enjoy a wider variety of dairy products. You can also buy lactose-free milk that has had lactase enzymes added to it to. Lactase enzymes digest the lactose, and then pasteurization neutralizes the lactase enzymes so they will not be active when you drink the milk.

If you think you may be lactose-intolerant, you can easily avoid lactose-induced digestive upset by avoiding dairy products highest in lactose, namely milk, cream, and cheese that has not been fermented, including farmer's cheese, string cheese, and mozzarella, as well as ricotta cheese, which is made from the lactose-rich whey portion of milk. Ice cream, pizza, cheese foods like nacho chips and dip, and Mexican foods often contain these kinds of dairy products and are important to avoid if you have lactose intolerance.

Lactose intolerance is less prevalent in geographic regions where dairy was consumed fresh. These are typically cold-climate locations, where fresh milk would ferment more slowly. Lactose intolerance is more prevalent in cultures where dairy was consumed after fermentation reduced or eliminated lactose sugar in milk. These are typically warmer-climate regions, including Africa and Asia, where fresh milk would ferment more quickly.

No matter your heritage, most people with lactose intolerance can actually eat fermented dairy such as low-sugar yogurt and hard cheeses like cheddar, Swiss, and provolone. Fermentation naturally reduces the lactose content because the microbes digest the sugar as they grow. In fact, the reason so many adults develop lactose intolerance has to do with the fact that traditionally most dairy was preserved not in refrigerators but by the process of fermentation, so most adults consumed their dairy after the lactose had been fermented away. Even butter can be cultured, and cultured butter is better for anyone with lactose intolerance. Other fermented dairy that might work for folks with lactose intolerance includes sour cream and Brie, while cream cheese is not fermented and will still contain a little bit, as with cream. Cottage cheese has only been fermented briefly, but some people with milder lactose intolerance can enjoy it.

PROBLEM: DIETARY RESTRICTIONS FOR GOUT, DIVERTICULITIS, OR KIDNEY STONES

My patients often report having been told by well-meaning medical specialists that they need to restrict their diet to prevent gout, diverticulitis, or kidney stones. The reality is there is little no evidence that any of these restrictions do anything other than restrict your access to necessary nutrients. The advice persists because it is based on ideas that seem to make sense when you only know a little bit about nutrition, as is the case with most physicians and dietitians. Without understanding that bad fats and excessive carbs disrupt metabolism, the foundation of standard nutrition advice is cracked and does far more harm than good.

That said, some people with gout, a disease where uric acid levels in the blood are elevated and uric acid stones form in your joints and cause episodic extreme pain, have noticed specific foods are triggers for their gout. If this is the case for you, continue avoiding the foods you've noticed trigger your gout, at least until your blood level of uric acid is reduced to normal.

With regard to kidney stone and gout prevention, most of my patients with either one of these problems tend to drink little water. If you have either condition, or are at risk of either due to medication use or family history, then I would strongly recommend making sure to get at least eight glasses (8 ounces) of water daily.

Turning to the issue of diverticulitis, next, quite a number of my patients who have had their first screening colonoscopy around age fifty were told they have diverticula in their colon, and need to restrict their diet to prevent infection. Diverticula are little pockets in the colon that are increasingly common as we age. Only 1 to 2 percent of children have them, but by age eighty, more than half the population has at least one. Patients with diverticula are sometimes told to avoid nuts and seeds and fruits with seeds (like strawberries) to prevent diverticulitis, a serious infection of those little pockets. But this advice is not based on any science whatsoever. Since most people with diverticula go through life not ever knowing they have them, much less that they're getting infections, it seems a little unwise to start telling folks to restrict their diets without any evidence to support the recommendation.

That said, a few of my patients unlucky enough to have chronic recurrences of diverticulitis have noticed specific foods trigger their diverticulitis, typically popcorn, nuts (but not nut butters), and lettuce. Very often, however, people have not had any of these foods and nevertheless get an infection. What typically triggers the diverticulitis in these cases is some kind of colonic irritation, like food poisoning, a flare of colitis, or an episode of constipation. If you have diverticulosis but have never had diverticulitis, there is no evidence that any dietary restriction is helpful and some evidence it can harm. If you have had diverticulitis, on the other hand, it's very important to prevent constipation and other sources of colonic irritation. Still, for most folks with asymptomatic diverticular disease, dietary restrictions should be considered experimental.

PROBLEM: PERSISTENT FATIGUE

If your fatigue is not something that goes away when you eat, I recommend you get a medical evaluation. If your doctor cannot find the cause, let's review a few common medications that may be making you tired.

Blood-Sugar-Lowering Medications

Insulin, glyburide, glipizide, and the "glitazones" can all push your blood sugar below your body's set point, particularly when you cut down on your carbohydrate intake. Dropping your blood sugar below where your brain wants it to be can cause fatigue, hypoglycemia, and weight gain. Make sure to work with your doctor to discuss this possibility, and any medication reduction you do should be closely monitored.

Cholesterol-Lowering Medications

In addition to causing hunger, cholesterol drugs can cause fatigue by several mechanisms.

First, they cause muscle pain, by blocking the ability of muscle cells to make the compounds muscle cells normally need to hold together. This causes microtears with activity and the healing process can be associated with fatigue. It also tends to make folks reluctant to engage in much activity. If you tell your doctor you're concerned that this may be the cause of your muscle aches, chances are he'll recommend a blood test for microtears (called "CK"), but the test is only positive in a tenth of the population with muscle damage. To make matters worse, some of the muscle damage is permanent, so stopping the drug won't necessarily make you feel better.

Second, cholesterol drugs can cause depression. Your brain is made of 15 percent cholesterol by weight, and these drugs reduce the cholesterol available to your brain. Without enough cholesterol, your neurons cannot easily make repairs, grow, form new memories, or release packages of feel-good chemicals like serotonin and dopamine into your synaptic cleft.

FREQUENTLY ASKED QUESTIONS

Are any artificial sweeteners safe?

Some seem to be, others are definitely not, and there's a middle ground as well.

First, the safe group. Stevia comes from a natural source and is minimally caloric. Monk fruit has a lot of potential, but it is relatively new and hasn't been studied as thoroughly as stevia. Allulose is another newcomer that has potential, but very little is known at this point.

The middle ground would be sugar alcohols, like erythritol and xylitol. These are not known to be toxic or carcinogenic, but may promote intestinal discomfort and brief headaches. If you don't get those problems from sugar alcohols, then they may be OK for you to use. I wouldn't recommend daily use, however, again due to limited information available on their long-term effects.

Sweeteners I'd avoid include the carcinogens sucralose, which was recently officially added to the list of carcinogens, and saccharin. I also recommend avoiding NutraSweet consumed in zero-calorie foods on an empty stomach because in these circumstances it can cross the blood-brain barrier in high enough concentration to promote migraines, a serious but reversible neurologic condition called transient global amnesia, and—in people prone to them—seizures.

Should I use an artificial sweetener?

They don't work for weight loss, but they may be useful for other purposes.

Every study on use of artificial sweeteners' ability to help people lose weight comes up showing that there is no benefit. Although in laboratory animals in controlled settings, some metabolic parameters do improve, when it comes to people living in the real world, these laboratory benefits evaporate. The problem with artificial sweeteners seems to be that they make you eat too much of the food you've just sweetened, just as sugar does, and ultimately you've gained little to nothing over simply using sugars.

This is why use of artificial sweeteners should be limited to helping you curb or cure a sweet tooth, by using them as a bridge at times where you really can't get sweetness without adding metabolism-disrupting amounts of sugar, as described in Chapter 12.

Doesn't exercise speed my metabolism?

No. Your metabolism does not speed up or slow down; it does not have "speeds." Your metabolism performs the tasks you ask of it. When you exercise, you burn more calories doing the work of exercising. Once you're done, you stop burning the extra calories and return to baseline. The literature out there showing that exercise builds muscle and then that muscle burns more calories for you while you are at rest does not really apply to anyone with normal muscle mass. For a non-bodybuilder to add a full pound of muscle can take months of dedicated exercise. The increase in calories burned by having that new pound of muscle is less than 10 per day. Exercise does help your health dramatically. But it's not an answer to weight control for most people who need to lose weight.

Don't I need to eat within thirty minutes after exercise to prevent muscle breakdown?

Here we have a perfect example of how sugar burners and fatburners live in different physiologic universes; rules that apply to one do not necessarily apply to the other.

If you are a sugar burner, it doesn't take a lot of intensity for your exercised muscles to produce an acid called pyruvate. Your muscles need to clear out this acid right away. Clearing out the acid forces your muscle to sacrifice some of its special amino acids, called branched-chain amino acids (BCAA). Without them, the muscle cell cannot rebuild itself properly after exercise. The result can be a net loss of muscle mass. So a sugar burner needs to eat more protein to prevent this loss of muscle. And not just any protein: proteins high in BCAAs.

When you're a fatburner, none of that stuff I just discussed applies to you. As your workouts don't produce anywhere near those levels of pyruvic acid, the clearing of this acid is not a major concern, and so your muscles don't need to use those very special BCAAs for that purpose. And since your building of muscle is a process that extends several days at least, there's no need to load up on protein, or anything else, right away. In fact, you're better off not eating immediately after a muscle-building workout. Exercise stimulates fat oxidation, i.e., burning fat, and waiting a while to eat after exercise will let you keep burning fat. If you eat, you've just wasted that metabolic boost. In other words, waiting to eat after exercise converts what was just a workout for your muscles into a workout for your metabolism as well.

This is another reason I don't strongly recommend starting a new exercise program until Phase II. If you are in the habit of exercising already, by all means continue.

Does my metabolism slow down when I get older?

No, but keep in mind that as you age, you also need fewer calories. So if it's been a few years since you last checked your daily calorie need, you should check in again. No matter how hard we train, we still lose lean tissue. The distribution of fat under our skin becomes uneven, disappearing from many areas leading to the appearance of piling up other odd places, but the reality is we actually can maintain a healthy, lower percentage of total body fat as we get older.

My cholesterol went up following this plan. Is that a problem?

No. In fact, if it goes up while your triglycerides go down, then that may mean you're burning body fat. After the liver picks up body fat released into your blood, it makes a short-lived particle called VLDL. VLDL turns into longer-lived LDL, which often goes up when you start to burn body fat.

As you read earlier, cholesterol does not damage your arteries. It's the inflammatory vegetable oils that disrupt the flow of cholesterol and fat-rich lipoproteins through your bloodstream, causing them to deposit on your arteries, which leads to heart attacks and strokes. Smoking disrupts the flow of these particles as well, which is why smokers have more heart attacks and strokes than nonsmokers. High blood sugar levels worsen the disruptions. Since the Fatburn Fix teaches you how to reduce high blood sugar and avoid vegetable oil, if your cholesterol level goes up while following the plan, it is highly unlikely to cause you any trouble. Especially if you don't smoke.

What does matter is the level of triglyceride, and usually people following the program see their triglyceride levels drop, which is a good thing.

Isn't dairy inflammatory?

No. Dairy is the only food designed by nature to be nourishing. It is not inflammatory, or mammals of earth would cease to exist.

Some people are allergic to dairy, and dairy is a common allergy trigger. But so are eggs, soy, wheat, peanuts, tree nuts, cats, dogs, horses, bees, pollen, grass, latex, and many other substances. When someone has an allergy, it is not a sign that whatever they're allergic to is toxic. It is a sign that they have an immune system that is reacting to the compound in a way that is not beneficial. The problem is the immune system, not the compound.

Some people are sensitive to the hormones in dairy and develop breast cysts or cystic acne. This is sometimes alleviated by getting organic dairy. Such cyst reactions may indicate you are exposed to high amounts of fluoride, since some of fluoride's ill effects are mediated through disruptions in hormone receptor function. Fluoride levels are surprisingly high in a lot of herbal, green, and black teas, so if you drink tea and have a problem with dairy, the problem may not be the dairy as much as the excessive fluoride.

Another consideration if you get cystic acne or problematic breast cysts is iodine deficiency, which can make you more sensitive to the effects of fluoride. (Iodine deficiency can also be a cause of breast cysts and acne regardless of dairy intake.)

Isn't gluten inflammatory?

No. Like dairy, wheat has long been maligned for one reason or another, and lately the rationale is based on research showing that a component of gluten called gliadin stimulates a compound the body makes, called zonulin, to allow white blood cells to move between cells of the intestine. This finding has led some to speculate that they've found the smoking gun proving gluten causes celiac disease, and possibly all manner of other autoimmune disease.

However this is not rational. The research does not support causation. It is merely a description of one step in the mechanism by which gliadin triggers an immune response. There is no research on the zonulin response to any other plant protein aside from the components of gluten, and now that nearly every component of gluten has been tested and shown to cause some degree of zonulin response, one might more rationally suppose that many proteins do the exact same thing as gluten. It may be that many proteins in the intestinal tract stimulate the body to release zonulin. This may be a normal and necessary reaction that has become exaggerated in folks with celiac disease. To suggest that gliadin-binding zonulin means that gliadin *causes* celiac is illogical, although sadly I have seen over three hundred articles in which researchers jumping on this bandwagon make that same logical error. It's illogical in the same way that it would be illogical to blame fires on fire engines just because they show up whenever there's a fire in town.

People with celiac disease, like all people with autoimmune diseases, have an immune system dysfunction. The root of their problem is not gluten. The root of celiac disease is dysfunction in the immune system that makes people with celiac respond abnormally to gluten. As long as you don't have celiac disease, you can enjoy your sprouted grain bread in peace.

What should I eat for bone health?

If you want to be a good fatburner, you do need to be active, and to be active, you need healthy bones. Your bones need more than just calcium; they also need magnesium, selenium, iodine, and vitamins A, D, and K2, along with protein. I recommend supplementing with vitamin D, since our body makes D only when our skin is exposed to sun, but most people get very little sunlight and very few foods are good sources of D. I also recommend supplementing with magnesium, since it's difficult for most people to eat enough on a normal diet given our depleted soil. Although minerals can be lost in the water if boiled or in the oil if fried, they are not typically damaged by cooking, so raw and cooked versions of the foods below will have about the same amounts of calcium (and the same is true for other minerals we will discuss). Here are foods that will help to supply you with each of the other bone-fortifying nutrients.

Calcium

Get at least three servings daily from the following calcium-rich foods (listed with serving size).

- American cheese: 1 ounce
- Almonds: 1¼ cups
- Beans, white: 1½ cups
- Broccoli: 8 cups chopped raw
- Cottage cheese: 12 ounces
- Hard cheeses (e.g., cheddar, swiss, provolone) and mozzarella: 1½ ounces
- Kale: 10 cups chopped raw
- Milk: 8 ounces
- Salmon, bone in: 3½ ounces
- Sardines, bone in: 1 can
- Tofu: 6 ounces firm (some tofu is fortified with calcium and contains twice the normal amount—check the nutrition label)
- Yogurt: 8 ounces

Selenium

The easiest way to get enough selenium is to eat one Brazil nut each week, or four per month. Too many may actually cause selenium toxicity. Other selenium-rich foods include:

- Halibut, cooked, 3 ounces: 47 mcg (67% DV)
- Sardines, canned, 3 ounces: 45mcg (64% DV)
- Grass-fed beef, cooked, 3 ounces: 33 mcg (47% DV)

- Turkey, cooked boneless, 3 ounces: 31 mcg (44% DV)
- Beef liver, cooked, 3 ounces: 28 mcg (40% DV)
- Chicken, cooked, 3 ounces: 22 mcg (31% DV)
- Egg, 1 large: 15 mcg (21% DV)
- Spinach, 1 cup: 11 mcg (16% DV)

Iodine

The easiest way to get enough iodine is to chew on a leaf of dulse seaweed every day, or otherwise finish off an ounce each week. One ounce of dulse seaweed has 770 percent DV. (It tastes perfect with an Asian-style salad—snip it into pieces with cooking shears.) Other iodine-rich foods include:

- Cod, cooked, 3 ounces: 99 mcg (66% DV)
- Yogurt, plain, 1 cup: 75 mcg (50% DV)
- Milk, whole, 1 cup: 56 mcg (37% DV)
- Egg, 1 large: 24 mcg (16% DV)
- Lima beans, cooked, 1 cup: 16 mcg (10% DV)

Vitamin K2

Vitamin K1 helps to clot your blood. Vitamin K2 was recognized less than a generation ago, and helps to direct calcium to your bones and teeth, which prevents it from ending up hardening your arteries or forming kidney stones and bone spurs. The recommended daily value has not been determined yet. K2 is a fat-soluble vitamin, so we have to eat fat to get it. It comes primarily from pasture-fed animals and from fermented foods. A good resource for more information on this just-discovered vitamin is *Vitamin K2 and the Calcium Paradox: How a Little-Known Vitamin Could Save Your Life*. Foods rich in vitamin K2 include:

- Natto (a certain type of fermented soy that tastes OK with lots of soy sauce—some Japanese people love it)
- Gouda cheese
- Hard cheese from cows raised on pasture
- Blue cheese
- Egg yolk

- Butter from cows raised on pasture
- Chicken liver
- Salami
- Chicken breast
- Ground beef

Vitamin A

Although we talk about plant sources of vitamin A, technically plants only provide vitamin A precursors (like retinoids) that our body converts to true vitamin A. Only animal products contain true vitamin A. I'm going to include both plants rich in vitamin A precursors and animal-derived foods rich in true vitamin A in this list.

- Butternut squash, cubed and cooked, 1 cup: 22,869 IU (457% DV)
- Kale, chopped, 1 cup: 10,302 IU (206% DV)
- Carrots, raw, 1 medium: 10,190 IU (204% DV)
- Beef liver, cooked, 1 ounce: 8,881 IU (178% DV)
- Spinach, raw, 1 cup: 2,813 IU (56% DV)
- Broccoli, raw, 1 cup: 567 IU (11% DV)
- Butter, 1 tablespoon: 350 IU (7% DV) (grass-fed has more)
- Egg, 1 large: 245 IU (5% DV)

Protein

More than 90 percent of the dry weight of your bones is protein, and inadequate dietary protein is one of the underappreciated causes of low bone density and weak bones. Although some folks going keto really keep their protein low, I don't recommend going below 60 grams for women or 80 for men. For a tool to estimate your protein intake, see the appendix.

How fast should I lose weight?

This depends largely on your Fatburn Quotient (see Chapter 9). The lower your score, the less ready you are to focus on weight loss. The higher your score, the more you can safely cut calories and be sure to burn fat and not burn muscle or lose bone mass, or stress your body's organs. Once your Fatburn Quotient is over 75, or you've been able to skip a meal without experiencing any of the hunger-emergency symptoms on the Hypo-glycemia Frequency Assessment worksheet, you're ready to focus on faster weight loss.

The rapidity of weight loss also depends on how much weight you've got to lose and how much you've already lost. If you've got 200 pounds to lose, you can drop 80 fairly quickly—in as little as six months if you're skipping meals frequently. But at some point things will plateau and you may need to give your body time to sort out the new situation. The part of your brain that gauges your fat mass and your muscle mass to decide if you are starving or well-fed needs to come to grips with the fact that there is much less of you than there was not too long ago, and sometimes it needs you to sit and coast for a few months or even a year at your new significantly reduced weight before it will be convinced that further weight loss is a good idea.

This is yet another reason why it's important for you to focus on how you feel, on how much energy you have, and how much you enjoy the taste of real food and the newfound freedom from dependence on processed food, energy drinks, and sugar. Celebrate the weight you've lost and the health you've gained. Enjoy the feeling of being energized and mentally sharp. Focus not on what you haven't yet accomplished, but on what your body can now do that it couldn't before. Focus not just on body composi-tion, but also on living life to its fullest.

I appreciate that this isn't the kind of language one typically runs into in a diet book where the selling point is radically fast weight loss and the downside of that approach is never considered.

You know the downsides. If you've only understood half of the concepts in the book, you're miles ahead of your doctor's understanding of weight loss and what differentiates healthy metabolic rehabilitation from a tem-porary drop in dress size. Between you and your doctor, you are now the expert in the room (on this topic at least).

Let me prove it: You've no doubt heard of drugs like Boniva and Fos-amax meant to slow or reverse the process of osteoporosis—thinning bone. When you think of osteoporosis, you not only think of weakened, hollowed-out bone, but also of a higher likelihood of a *fragility fracture* that can be significant enough to affect your ability to move about without pain for the rest of your life. You know that healthy, youthful bones are less likely to break, and so if these drugs can rejuvenate bone, who wouldn't be pushing their way to the front of the line to be sure to receive one?

The fact is, these drugs work by preventing your body from reabsorbing old worn-out bone material in a hip, say, or your spine, thus making it appear that your bones are stronger than they really are. That old worn-out bone contains calcium, which is what bone-density tests measure, and so the drugs increase the total amount of calcium in bone. That's how bone-density drugs make your bones appear strong when in fact they are more prone to breaking than they would be otherwise.

Here's the thing: there's a reason your bones reabsorb aged bone material. It's because it's riddled with microfractures that are invisible to the eye, like a bridge that looks structurally sound from a distance but upon closer examination is revealed to be so rusted it is at the edge of catastrophic failure. If you follow the metaphor, taking drugs that make your bones *look* better is as useful as painting the bridge. It looks as good as new, but you probably don't want to drive across it. Paint doesn't hold up bridges—we know this intuitively, and every engineer will agree with this.

But not every doctor knows that losing weight without correcting the underlying metabolic disorders that block your fatburn is as futile as painting bridges. And saying that some new fad fast-weight-loss diet—without any underlying science to buttress it—is the one that will finally work is as ridiculous as if some self-appointed expert jumps up and suggests that the reason the rusted-out but brightly painted bridges are falling down is that we're using the wrong paint. There is a science to the building and maintenance of a bridge that is structurally sound and safe for one to cross. And likewise, there is a science to metabolic rehabilitation and the stages you must progress through to restore your fatburn systems—and the rest of your body—to health.

But of course, you now know all this, don't you? And now you know what to do about it.

Epilogue

In 2013, just about a week before the NBA All-Star break, my husband, Luke, and I were watching a Lakers game when we both noticed something un- usual about seven-foot "Superman" center Dwight Howard's play. When he leapt up to grab a rebound off the rim, the ball simply bounced off his hands.

I'd witnessed this kind of sloppy ball handling all week. It was as if he were wearing oven mitts. I'd also heard an interview a few weeks prior where he was complaining about tingling in his feet after a recent back surgery. I suspected he also had tingling in his fingertips because I knew that a diet like his, which included every manner of junk food, loaded with vegetable oil and sugar, would set him up for nerve damage and symptoms similar to carpal tunnel. Unlike with carpal tunnel, however, the symptoms were not limited to his hands.

Now that you've read this book, I hope you understand that nerve dam- age is just one of many metabolic consequences of the kind of diet that dis- rupts fatburn, and therefore you already know it would likely be reversed by a diet that revives fatburn—even in a person of normal weight.

What made it particularly likely that Howard's symptoms resulted from metabolic disruptions (and not the back surgery itself) was the fact that his diet was especially unhealthy. First, he was eating a lot of sugar—the equiva- lent of twenty-four Hershey's bars a day, as would later be reported by ESPN and other news outlets—and so that's the part of the diet that got the most attention. What the reporters didn't say, because it complicated the story, was that our intervention didn't involve merely yanking the candy from his hands. It was an extreme diet makeover that ensured adaptation of the five rules you're now familiar with, starting with the most important: eliminating vegetable oils from his diet, and including only clean-burning fats, along with the other rules you've read about: to seek salt, drink water, and supplement with vitamins, minerals, and superfoods. Taking these five steps put him on a path to reversing the damage in all four of his fatburn systems.

And now that you've finished this book, I hope you can predict what happened next. With a personal chef and team of assistants to help, Howard's improved metabolism generated headline-grabbing improvements in performance: "Superman Returns!" In a series of interviews that followed the All-Star break, Howard repeatedly attributed the miraculous turnaround to his new diet.

Over the ensuing months, as he continued to follow the five rules, his four fatburn systems continued to recover. Some of the effects were entirely predictable, including more energy; some less so, including a shoulder MRI showing previously torn cartilage had spontaneously healed to the point surgery was no longer indicated. Subsequent lab work showed that not only was Howard performing better, so was every cell in his body; his metabolism had been revitalized. And once your fatburn systems recover, you too will experience dramatic improvements—improved energy, reduced inflammation, better moods, better digestion, better sleep, and so on—whether you start to lose weight right away or not.

How had I finally convinced Howard to change his eating habits?

At Luke's suggestion, I'd used a scary-sounding medical term: "dysesthesia." "I don't want *that*," I remember him saying in his soft Georgia drawl. But that's not what clinched it. What sealed the deal was me putting skin in the game, saying to Howard in plain terms, "Let me change your diet. Do what I ask, and I promise you will see significant improvement in your back pain, your tingling, and your energy in two weeks or I'll leave my position with the Lakers because that would mean I don't know what the heck I'm talking about." That's how sure I was that this was going to work.

That's the same message I want to leave with you. This is going to work.

Dwight Howard was in a place of professional crisis. But he decided to trust me for no other reason than the fact that what I was telling him made sense: even though his weight was normal, his metabolism was not. His body was failing to heal on a diet comprised of inhuman amounts of junk foods, loaded with sugar and vegetable oil—levels of toxin that effectively undermined the positive effects of any good food he was getting. He hadn't been told what you now know: when you're eating junk food—whether in the form of chips or fast-food fries or the thousands of convenience foods sold to us as healthy (due to low saturated fat content)—you're eating unhealthy volumes of toxic oil. Like most athletes and most of my patients, whether overweight or not, he'd never heard that vegetable oils could disrupt if not entirely derail an athletic career. And he had no idea he was on the fast track to developing other, additional complications of a metabolism disrupted enough to place him on the diabetes spectrum.

I want to leave you with this last idea, a way to look at the relationship between metabolic health, fatburn, and diet: all (or nearly all) chronic diseases that doctors see and treat every day are manifestations of the reality that a person is developing diabetes. Whether you have been officially diagnosed with diabetes or not, if you have suffered a heart attack, needed a stent, suffer from migraines, any psychiatric condition, autoimmunity, multiple sclerosis, Parkinson's or Alzheimer's, even cancer, you are somewhere on the diabetes spectrum. And that means you have more control over your own health destiny than you've been told.

I caught Howard's attention by putting my reputation at stake. I intend to do that again here, with this book. I believe, as firmly as I have believed anything in my medical career, that if you take the five steps outlined in this book, you can restore your fatburn and normalize your blood sugar. In doing so you'll be getting off the diabetes spectrum and improving or even recovering completely from chronic diseases that you may be suffering from now, while simultaneously making yourself powerfully resistant to developing other serious conditions in the future.

Small steps, repeated often, can lead to massive health improvements over time. Even if you only eliminate the vegetable oils and can't take the other four steps that are part of the Fatburn Fix Plan, you will be clearing the way for vast health improvements.

Were this a courtroom (held in an unlikely spot, right in the front of a grocery store), I would point to the aisles of junk food and call the worst enemies of your health out by name: canola, corn, cottonseed, soy, sunflower, safflower, grapeseed, and rice bran. As far as I am concerned, these uber-processed oils stand against everything I stand for as a physician. The sad fact is that these oils are everywhere. The more you look, the more you'll find. And we're all eating them, even when we don't know it. That's exactly as the food manufacturers would have it, as well as the "health" conglomerates, and all those who live in a bigger house as a direct benefit of the fact that they've been making you and your family sick.

I hope that with this book I've put skin in the game. I'm saying that if you get vegetable oil out of your diet, it *will* make a difference. You'll feel it in your body. You'll see it in your lab results—and in the mirror. And I am certain that the same principle applies nationwide. If we eat more vegetable oil, we're going to get sicker, and if we eat less, our health will improve; these things are connected. If we hope for the people around us to become healthier, we must first become healthy ourselves and then spread the good news. It's really not that radical of an idea: identify those things that characterize junk food and then get them out of your diet. The key dietary claim I'm making is that the central defining feature of junk food is the inclusion of vegetable oils, which are toxic to the body.

If you are convinced by the arguments I've made, you are not alone. There are growing numbers of chefs, nutritionists, naturopaths, osteopaths, dietitians, medical doctors, chiropractors, physical therapists, respiratory therapists, athletic trainers, athletes, social workers, biohackers, podcasters, journalists, educators, moms, military, and other public servants who all just want to eat real food that gives our bodies a chance to be energized, to feel healthy, and to allow us to do the things we want to do in this precious time we have on earth.

Vegetable oil is not a part of that happy story—that's my claim. If you do nothing more than make a conscious effort to get these oils out of your life, you are going to feel better. And when you do, I ask only that you spread the good word. If you've lost weight, have more energy, and start to look younger, try not to keep it a secret. Eat as if your body is starving for a connection to the natural world. That connection is most powerfully created by eating intensely flavorful, fresh ingredients raised in healthy soil.

When you celebrate good food, you are celebrating your body. Believe this as if your life depends on it.

Acknowledgments

First and foremost, Dado and Steve, Super Agents at Folio Lit, who inspired and supported me from the genesis of this book and through all its transformations. And many thanks to my editor, Sarah Murphy, for gently nurturing this project to maturity and finding the best path forward.

I am especially grateful to filmmaker Jeff Hayes, who has supported the message of *Deep Nutrition* since the early days and has introduced me to amazing people over the years who also believe in the message. Without Jeff's support, this book would probably not have happened. I am also indebted to support from podcast luminaries including Dave Asprey, Brad Kearns, Mark Sisson, David Perlmutter, M.D., Joe Mercola, M.D., Vinnie Tortorich, Adam Corolla, Drew Pinsky, M.D., Sean Stevenson, Katie Wells, Jimmy Moore, Abel James, Ben Greenfeld, Sean Croxton, Diane Sanfilippo, and Liz Wolfe.

Much of this book was originally created as a resource for team members at ABC Fine Wine and Spirits, and I am forever indebted to the executive leadership team and the board members who made the bold decision to bring a doctor on board to serve the 1,600 plus people employed at ABC. And nobody deserves more thanks than Charlie Bailes IV, who had the original vision of hiring me and is still crazy enough to work toward changing the world for the better.

Finally, to my wonderful husband Luke, for always believing in me.

Resources

There's a war being waged over your food choices. If you want to learn more about the winners and losers in the nutrition science wars, it's now easier than ever, as concerned physicians are finally able to get the word out. Here are a few of my favorite examples:

CANCER

Cancer: A Metabolic Disease with Metabolic Solutions
www.youtube.com/watch?v=SEE-oU8_NSU

Cancer as a Mitochondrial Metabolic Disease
www.youtube.com/watch?v=KusaU2taxow

Cancer Is Not Genetic
This lecture at the National Institutes of Health highlights the role of mitochondrial dysfunction—such as that brought on by a diet high in vegetable oil—in causing cancer as well as many diseases associated with premature aging.
www.youtube.com/watch?v=xDDFV7Sovvs

Diet and Cancer
Dr. Thomas Seyfried is the world's leading authority on the role of diet in producing cancer. The following two lectures provide a fascinating summary of his more recent work:

Fasting Glucose Is a Risk Factor for Breast Cancer
cebp.aacrjournals.org/content/11/11/1361

High Blood Sugar Linked to Cancer Risk
www.webmd.com/cancer/news/20070227/high-blood-sugar-linked-cancer
-risk#1

Starving Cancer by Depriving It of Sugar: Dr. Sophia Lunt
www.youtube.com/watch?v=f6rSuJ2YheQ&t=52s

Starving Cancer with Dr. Dominic D'Agostino
www.youtube.com/watch?v=oUP9fFUi7lE

CHOLESTEROL

Are Cholesterol Pills Safe?
This study shows that taking cholesterol-lowering drugs (statins) offers no benefits
for people over 65 who do not already have heart disease. In fact, taking statins may
even shorten lives.
jamanetwork.com/journals/jamainternalmedicine/fullarticle/2628971?

Correcting Four Decades of the Wrong Dietary Advice
journals.lww.com/jaapa/Fulltext/2016/07000/Correcting_four_decades_of_the
_wrong_dietary.14.aspx

Heart of the Matter
Part Two of a program from the award-winning news show *Catalyst* (think of it as an
Australian version of *60 Minutes*) exposing the controversial use of statins and the
moneyed interests that pay for science. The show first aired in 2013.
www.youtube.com/watch?v=5ZvvGPN5glY

Heart of the Matter: The Inside Story
A presentation by the acclaimed Australian journalist who led the investigation into
the above news story.
www.youtube.com/watch?v=BzTjPuikhQE&t=34s

Re-evaluation of the Traditional Diet-Heart Hypothesis
This article provides analysis of recovered data from Minnesota Coronary Experiment (1968-73).
www.bmj.com/content/353/bmj.i1246

A Rigorous Assessment of the Myth that Cholesterol Causes Heart Disease

The hypothesis that cholesterol causes heart disease is dead. Listen carefully as David Diamond, Ph.D., shreds this hypothesis, and the drug-company sponsored "research" that "proved" it to be true. At the end of the video he explains very clearly what the research shows and explains very clearly who should, and who should not, take a cholesterol/LDL lowering drug.

www.youtube.com/watch?v=hCvlvu_Ssw4

An Update on Demonization and Deception in Research on Saturated Fat

For the past 60 years there has been a concerted effort to demonize saturated fats, found in animal products and tropical oils, and the cholesterol in our food and blood. Despite the well-established health benefits of diets rich in cholesterol and saturated fat, flawed, deceptive, and biased research has created the myth that a low fat, plant-based diet is ideal for good health.

www.youtube.com/watch?v=uc1XsO3mxX8

What Your Doctor Doesn't Know About Saturated Fat

drcate.com/what-every-doctor-should-know-about-ancel-keys-experiments

DOCTORS TO FOLLOW

Dr. Eric Berg (Chiropractic Doctor)
www.youtube.com/channel/UC3w193M5tYPJqF0Hi-7U-2g

Ken Berry, M.D.
www.youtube.com/channel/UCIma2WOQs1Mz2AuOt6wRSUw

Georgia Ede, M.D.
www.diagnosisdiet.com

Andreas Einfelt, M.D.
www.dietdoctor.com

Jason Fung, M.D.
www.youtube.com/watch?v=jXXGxoNFag4&t=826s

Sarah Halberg, M.D.
www.youtube.com/watch?v=ESL3_7sdCwU

Tro Kalayjian, M.D.
www.doctortro.com

EVENTS AND MEETINGS

These are organized events for doctors, health enthusiasts, thought leaders, and health seekers who congregate to share real science (not fake news):

KetoCon
www.ketocon.org/about-us

Keto Mojo
These makers of reliable blood ketone test meters maintain an exceptional resource for many more meetings.
keto-mojo.com/keto-low-carb-events

Low Carb Down Under
lowcarbdownunder.com.au

Low Carb USA
www.lowcarbusa.org

ONLINE SUPPORT GROUPS WITH SIMILAR DIET PHILOSOPHIES

Dirty Lazy Keto
www.facebook.com/groups/dirtylazyketo

Keto Connect
www.facebook.com/ketoconnect2

LCHF Low Carb High Fat
www.facebook.com/groups/LCHF4LIFE

GOOD FATS

Traditionally Used Fats and Oils
Flavorful, minimally processed, and unrefined

All Purpose	Caution with Heat
Olive oil	Walnut oil
Avocado oil	Flax oil
Peanut oil	Sesame
Butter/Ghee	Walnuts
Tallow & Lard	Seeds
Cocoa Butter	Fatty Fish
Mac Nut oil	Artisanal grapeseed
Coconut oil	
Almond oil	
Unrefined Palm	
Palm Kernel oil	© DrCate.com

OK BUT NOT SO GREAT

Refined Traditional Fats (Label Says "Refined")

Refined Avocado, Refined Coconut,
Refined Palm, Refined Peanut

BAD FATS

ALWAYS read ingredients list before buying ANY
packaged goods to avoid the bad oils:

Name of Oil	Common Products Containing Bad Oils
Canola oil	Fake whip cream
Corn oil	Fake butter spreads
Cottonseed oil	Margarine
Safflower oil	Vegetable shortening
Soy oil	Store-bought pastries
Sunflower oil	Chicken nuggets
Hydrogenated oil	Restaurant fried foods
Vegetable oil	Most chips & crackers
	Most protein bars
Mostly in Restaurants:	Most salad dressings
Grapeseed oil	Most mayo brands
Ricebran oil	Most granola & cereal
"Blended" olive oils	Most dips & spreads

PHASE I ACCELERATED LUNCH MENU

TUNA or EGG SALAD (no bread)	• 1-3 eggs, 1-2 Tbsp cooking fat, optional bacon/sausage/herbs/veg
MASON JAR SALAD	• Layered salad marinade in a Mason jar, keeps for days in the fridge
WRAP 'n' ROLL	• Your favorite deli meat wrapped with your favorite cheese & more
DO-IT-YOURSELF INSTANT SOUP	• Add a few ready-to-eat ingredients to a good, flavorful stock
KETO CRUST PIZZA	• Same as Phase I but instead of flour dough buy cauliflower crust
WATER	• Aids digestion, especially important for high protein/high fat foods
BULLETPROOF COFFEE	• Same as Chapter 12
REAL FOOD PROTEIN SHAKE	• Swap out the powder for real-food protein sources (see Chapter 12)

About the Author

Dr. Cate trained in biochemistry and genetics at Cornell University before attending Robert Wood Johnson Medical School. Practicing in Hawaii she discovered that her older patients who grew up eating traditional foods were healthier than their own children and realized that most of what dietitians and doctors learn about nutrition is dangerously wrong. She is the author of several books, including the underground classic *Deep Nutrition* and *Food Rules*. She designed a nutritional plan for the LA Lakers, which has been duplicated by the Wizards, Villanova Basketball, and dozens of amateur and professional sports teams, and she currently works with professional athletes to optimize their metabolism for energy and performance. She also directs a corporate metabolic health program for one of Florida's largest family-owned companies. She has been featured in several documentary films and major media outlets, including *Sports Illustrated, Vogue, Prevention, Reader's Digest*, the *New York Post*, and the *Los Angeles Times*, as well as on numerous TV and radio shows and podcasts. She lives in Florida with her husband, Luke, a German shephard, and a Maine coon. Follow Dr. Cate at DrCate.com.